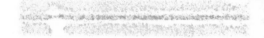

THE HEALTH PSYCHOLOGY

OF WOMEN

Edited by

Catherine A. Niven

and

Douglas Carroll
Glasgow Polytechnic, UK

Switzerland • Australia • Belgium • France • Germany • Great Britain
India • Japan • Malaysia • Netherlands • Russia • Singapore • USA

Harwood Academic Publishers

Private Bag 8
Camberwell, Victoria 3124
Australia

3-14-9, Okubo
Shinjuku-ku, Tokyo 169
Japan

58, rue Lhomond
75005 Paris
France

Emmaplein 5
1075 AW Amsterdam
Netherlands

Glinkastrasse 13–15
O-1086 Berlin
Germany

820 Town Center Drive
Langhorne, Pennsylvania 19047
United States of America

Post Office Box 90
Reading, Berkshire RG1 8JL
Great Britain

Library of Congress Cataloging-in-Publication Data

The Health psychology of women/edited by Catherine A. Niven and
  Douglas Carroll.
    p. cm.
  Includes bibliographical references and index.
  ISBN 3-7186-5335-4 (hard).—ISBN 3-7186-5336-2 (soft)
  1. Women—Health and hygiene. 2. Women—Mental health.
3. Clinical health psychology. I. Niven, Catherine, A.
II. Carroll, Douglas.
  [DNLM: 1. Women—psychology. 2. Women's Health. WA 300 H43397]
RA564.85.H433 1992
613'.0424'019—dc20
DNLM/DLC
for Library of Congress   92-49332
                                           CIP

Catherine A. Niven
to Seonaid and her baby, my first grandchild, as yet unborn;
may they be healthy

Douglas Carroll
to Anne, for buffering the worst of life's stresses

CONTENTS

PREFACE

Inequalities in health are well recognized. These are most obvious when one compares the health of those living in Third World countries with those living in the so-called "developed" First World. Even within Western countries, however, health inequalities exist between the rich and the poor, the dominant and minority ethnic populations. They are also apparent between men and women. At first glance it is men who appear to be at a disadvantage since the male death rate exceeds the female death rate from conception to old age. Thus we might wish to recognize and celebrate the ability of women to survive. However, surviving has a price—women have much higher rates of mental and physical illness than men, hence the maxim "men die, but women suffer".

Since health psychology is concerned with psychological aspects of life and death, well-being and suffering, it might be expected that its researchers would be keen to examine psychological aspects of male *and* female experience as they relate to health and that health psychology would be at the forefront of the debate surrounding gender differences in this context. Sadly health psychology research has followed health research in being mainly concerned with men. Except in the area of reproductive psychology which focuses predominantly, but not exclusively on women, health psychology has a bias towards using male subjects and studying 'male' diseases (i.e., those that kill more men than women) and male health promotion. It is this layer of inequality which this book seeks to redress.

We would like to express our gratitude to our many colleagues within and without Glasgow Polytechnic who have stimulated our thoughts and clarified our ideas. Our students have occasionally moderated our enthusiasms and brought us down to earth. Essential practical support and assistance has been, as always, provided by Mrs Catherine Wright. Finally, we would like to thank the contributors to this text for their enthusiasm and encouragement.

CONTRIBUTORS

Elizabeth Alder, PhD

Elizabeth Alder is lecturer in health psychology at Queen Margaret College, Edinburgh, UK. She has a first degree in psychology and a doctorate in animal behavior. She teaches health psychology to health professionals and is active in research on reproductive health. She is secretary of the Psychobiology Section of the British Psychological Society and was founding chair of the Society of Reproductive and Infant Psychology. She has three teenage daughters and is optimistic about the opportunity for reproductive choices for women in the next generation.

Barbara L. Andersen, PhD

Barbara Andersen is a professor in the Departments of Psychology, and of Obstetrics and Gynecology at the Ohio State University, in Columbus, USA. Her main research interests include female sexuality, psychological aspects of cancer and cancer treatment, and psychological interventions to enhance the quality of life.

John Bancroft, MD

John Bancroft is a clinical consultant in the MRC Reproductive Biology Unit and honorary senior lecturer in the University Department of Psychiatry, Edinburgh, UK. He obtained his MD from the University of Cambridge and is a fellow of the Royal Colleges of Physicians of London, and Edinburgh, and of the Royal College of Psychiatrists. His main research interests are the relationship between reproductive hormones, mood and behavior, and the psychosomatic determinants of male sexual dysfunction.

Alan J. Blair, PhD

Alan Blair is an honorary research fellow at the University of Birmingham, UK, where he undertook post-doctoral research into the interpersonal and intrapersonal dynamics underlying individuals' eating behavior. He is also presently completing a training course in clinical psychology at the University of Leicester. Additional interests include the role of primary prevention.

George R. Brown, MD

George Brown is senior research scientist for the Behavioral Medicine Research Program, Henry M. Jackson Foundation for the Advancement of Military Medicine, Maryland, and clinical associate professor of psychiatry at the University of Texas Health Science Center and the Uniformed Services University of the Health Sciences, USA. He initiated the first prospective study of psychiatric conditions in early stage HIV disease in women in the US, now in its fifth year of follow-up.

Douglas Carroll, PhD

Douglas Carroll is currently professor of psychology and head of the Department of Psychology at Glasgow Polytechnic, UK. He has researched and written widely on health psychology issues, in particular the role of psychological stress and behavior in cardiovascular disease.

Raymond Cochrane, PhD

Raymond Cochrane is a professor of psychology and dean of the Faculty of Science at the University of Birmingham, UK. His main research interests concern social factors in mental illness and the processes of immigrant adjustment.

Karel Gijsbers, PhD

Karel Gijsbers is a lecturer in physiological psychology at Stirling University, UK. His first degree was in physics. Subsequently he "converted" to psychology and obtained his PhD from McGill University, Montreal, Canada. His research interests include labor pain and pain in athletes.

Susan S. Girdler, PhD

Susan Girdler is currently clinical assistant professor of psychology in the Department of Psychiatry at the University of California at San Francisco (Fresno Division), USA. Dr Girdler's doctoral dissertation research (completed in 1991) centered on gender and female reproductive hormones as modulators of cardiovascular stress responses. Her current research addresses the independent and interactive effects of nicotine and oral contraceptive use on cardiovascular responses of young women.

Michele Goldschmidt, MS

Michele Goldschmidt is research associate for the Behavioral Medicine Research Program, Henry M. Jackson Foundation for the Advancement of Military Medicine, Maryland, USA. She has been involved in women's health issues for several years and is currently completing her dissertation examining health care provider-initiated discussions about HIV/AIDS during routine gynecological visits.

Cynthia Graham, PhD

Cynthia Graham is a research psychologist in the MRC Reproductive Biology Unit, Edinburgh, UK. She is currently working on a World Health Organization project investigating the effects of steroidal contraceptives on women's well-being and sexuality. She obtained an MAppSci in clinical psychology from the University of Glasgow and her PhD in clinical psychology from McGill University, Montreal, Canada. Her research interests include premenstrual changes, menstrual synchrony and the behavioral effects of oral contraceptives.

Marie Johnston, PhD

Marie Johnston is a professor in the Department of Psychology at the University of St Andrews, Scotland. She is president of the European Health Psychology Society and founder chair of the Health Psychology Section of the British Psychological Society. Her main research interests are responses to chronic and disabling diseases, and stress associated with medical procedures including gynaecological operations, prenatal testing and IVF.

Vivien J. Lewis, PhD

Vivien Lewis is Head of Adult Mental Health Psychology with the Mental Health Foundation of mid-Staffordshire and an Honorary Senior Research Fellow at the University of Birmingham. She has worked extensively, both clinically and in research, in the area of distress associated with food and body image. She also has a special interest in wider gender issues.

Kathleen A. Light, PhD

Kathleen Light is currently associate professor of psychology in the Department of Psychiatry at the University of North Carolina at Chapel Hill, USA. Dr Light has been active in research in the area of stress and the cardiovascular system since 1976.

Gillian McIlwaine, MD, PhD

Gillian McIlwaine is a consultant in public health medicine in the Greater Glasgow Health Board with a special responsibility for women's health. She graduated in medicine from the University of Aberdeen, UK. Her main interests have been in obstetrics and gynecology, in obstetric epidemiology, and the delivery of health care, and more recently in women's health in its widest context.

Catherine A. Niven, RGN, PhD

'Kate' Niven trained as a nurse and mothered two children before obtaining her first and higher degrees at the University of Stirling, UK. She currently lectures in developmental and health psychology at Glasgow Polytechnic. Her research interests include childbirth, prematurity, pain, and stress in carers.

David Sheffield, BSc

David Sheffield is a research student at Glasgow Polytechnic. His research interests are centered on the effects of social support on health, and he is currently working in this area for his PhD theses.

Lydia Temoshok, PhD

Lydia Temoshok is principal scientist and director of the Behavioral Medicine Research Program, Henry M. Jackson Foundation for the Advancement of Military

Medicine, Maryland, and associate professor in the Department of Psychiatry and the Neurosciences Program at the Uniformed Services University of the Health Sciences, USA. She is involved in pioneering work in the areas of HIV/AIDS, biopsychosocial oncology, psychoneuroimmunology, health psychology and behavioral medicine.

1

GENDER, HEALTH AND STRESS

DOUGLAS CARROLL AND CATHERINE A. NIVEN

Department of Psychology, Glasgow Polytechnic, Cowcaddens Road, Glasgow G4 0BA, UK

According to Matarazzo (1980), health psychology encompasses the total sum of the contributions that the discipline of psychology has to make to matters of health and well-being. The realms of contribution range from the etiological to the therapeutic; health psychology is concerned with untangling the psychological factors that contribute to health, to the onset and course of illness and disease and also with the application of psychological knowledge and techniques to the amelioration and prevention of illness and disease and the promotion of health.

Clearly health psychology has set itself an ambitious agenda for a project of recent vintage. In practice, though, health psychology has focused on more circumscribed areas than those defined above. Given such a broad brief, it is perhaps hardly surprising that some issues have occupied more attention than others. Particular areas of investment have been cardiovascular disease and cancer and more recently HIV and AIDS. This has lead some to object that, for the most part, the dominant preoccupation of health psychology has been with men and men's ailments. However, it is not just the selection of topic, but also the orientation toward it, that has fuelled this protest.

GENDER DIFFERENCES IN RESEARCH FOCUS

As Rodin and Ickovics (1990) pointed out, "White men continue to be almost exclusively studied in major health-care and pharmacological research. Even in animal-model research, male animals are almost always used" (Rodin and Ickovics, 1990, p. 1025). Examples are not hard to find. The Western Collaborative Group Study (Rosenman *et al.*, 1975) provided the stimulus for, as well as setting the tone of, much of the research into the relationship between heart disease and type A behaviour, a coping style characterized by competitive striving, time urgency and hostility. It involved a prospective investigation of over 3000 male, middle-aged non-manual workers. The subsequent Multiple Risk Factor Intervention Trial (Shekelle *et al*., 1985), which posed perhaps the greatest challenge to the type A concept was also directed exclusively toward men. Ninety percent of the subjects in the Recurrent Coronary Prevention Project (Friedman *et al*., 1986), which examined the impact of the psychological modification of type A behavior on the recurrence of heart disease, were men.

A number of justifications have been offered for this bias. In studies examining human cardiovascular reactions to psychological stress, women have, until recently, frequently been excluded on the grounds that their normal hormonal fluctuations might serve to contaminate results, rendering interpretation difficult. In the case of large scale intervention studies, the desire to protect women of child-bearing age from possible exposure to toxic substances or procedures has been cited, as has the additional cost of increasing the sample size by including women. However, undoubtedly the most consistently voiced justification for a male bias in the study of cardiovascular disease is men's substantially higher mortality rate.

It is true that in most Western countries the cardiovascular disease gender mortality ratio is 2:1 in women's favour, ie. that twice as many men die from heart disease as women. In terms of premature mortality, ie. in the age range 45–64, men's relative disadvantage is almost 3:1 (see, eg. Hart, 1989). However, there are compelling reasons for suspecting these various justifications as a sound basis for excluding women as subjects in the study of cardiovascular disease. First of all, research on the effects of women's hormonal status on cardiovascular reactions to psychological stress could contribute valuable information on the pathophysiology of cardiovascular disease. Secondly, as Rodin and Ickovics (1990) pointed out, while the protective policy of excluding women from health trials is almost certainly well-intentioned, there are groups of women, who, since they are at little or no risk of becoming pregnant, could easily be included. Finally, and most importantly, men's disadvantage in terms of cardiovascular disease mortality constitutes a poor justification for excluding women from study. After all, in most Western countries, cardiovascular disease is the leading cause of death for women as well as for men. Further, by studying women and cardiovascular disease, we may gain insight into what is affording women their protective advantage and this may yield dividends for both men and women.

Turning now to cancer, it again appears that women are under-represented in studies exploring possible psychological factors. Given that certain cancers are specific to women, we would anticipate that they might have attracted greater scrutiny in this context than with regard to cardiovascular disease. Nevertheless, although women have received somewhat more equitable study, large scale prospective investigations have tended to concentrate on men. For example, perhaps the largest prospective exploration to date of the contribution of psychological factors to cancer was the study conducted at Western Electric Company near Chicago (Persky *et al*., 1987). Its 2000 subjects were men. While the overall gender mortality ratios for cancer hover around 2:1 in women's favour, in most Western countries men and women register far less of a difference in the 45–64 age range. In fact, in some countries, eg. Sweden, the gender cancer mortality rates for this age range are almost equal. It is also perhaps worth noting that it is for cancers developing within this age range that psychological factors have been most implicated (eg. Fox, 1978).

Almost certainly, HIV and AIDS presents health psychology with one of its foremost challenges. However, its initial appearance in Western countries among homosexual and bisexual persons has tended to give a particular direction to psychological and biomedical research. Again, to date, men, mostly the white middle–class and middle–aged, have been the predominant focus of study. As Rodin and Ickovics (1990) attested, "beyond prevalence and basic epidemiology the issue of women and AIDS has received only limited research attention" (p. 1027). It remains the case that in both North America and Europe, AIDS continues to be far more common among men than women. However, the incidence of the disease among women is starting to rise sharply, as are estimates of their numbers infected with HIV. In the United States for example, the present rate of increase of AIDS in women is two and a half times that in men. In addition, around a third of women in Western countries have contracted AIDS through heterosexual intercourse, whereas the comparable statistic for men is under five percent.

Further, if we consider the epidemiology of AIDS in the area of its greatest prevalence, i.e. sub-Saharan Africa, a different gender distribution emerges. Since the mode of transmission in such countries has been almost exclusively that of heterosexual sexual intercourse, as many, if not more, women are affected as men. Chin (1990) estimates that some two and a half million women in sub-Saharan Africa had been infected by HIV by the end of the 1980s and that some quarter of a million had already developed AIDS.

Chin's projections for 1992 indicate the rate of spread of HIV and AIDS in sub-Saharan Africa. Some four million women were predicted to have been infected by the virus by then, and the cumulative AIDS total was predicted to be 600,000. Since the bulk of such women are, as in the case in Western countries, of child-bearing age, this clearly has massive implications for HIV infection and AIDS in children. While in the West we are only beginning to be confronted with the problem of children being infected with HIV prenatally from infected mothers, Chin reckoned that by the end of the 1980s HIV infection was the lot of some half a million African children and this figure was estimated to rise to one million by 1992. The corresponding figures for AIDS were 290,000 and 600,000 respectively. During the late 1980s in many central African cities, 5–10 percent of all infants were HIV positive. These figures not only give some idea of the pandemic character of the disease but also of its significance for women. In the West, where the resources that can be directed to biomedical and social psychological research are manifestly more substantial than those available in African countries, it is critical that the research focus shifts to incorporate the study of women.

GENDER DIFFERENCES IN MORTALITY AND MORBIDITY

From the foregoing, the reader will rightly infer that there are marked overall differences in the mortality rates of men and women in Western countries, which, to an extent, have directed the health psychology agenda. In almost every decade of life men die at a greater rate than women. If anything, these discrepancies in life expectancy in the West have increased in the last forty years, although there is evidence of at least some modest narrowing of the gap in some countries, eg. the US, in the last decade.

Nevertheless, according to the most current statistics (National Centre for Health Statistics, United States, 1989) life expectancy in the US is 71 years for men compared to 78 years for women, a seven-year advantage for women. In the UK (Office of Population Censuses and Surveys, 1989), the analogous figures are 72 and 78, an advantage of six years. Further, even in countries where male life expectancy is at the high end of the distribution, women still live longer. For example, in Japan male life expectancy in 1986 was 75 years; for Japanese females, though, it was 81 years (Marmot and Davey Smith, 1989).

In contrast, women have higher levels of morbidity than men. Morbidity simply refers to ill-health and almost every index of ill-health testifies that women suffer predominantly more than men: women consult physicians more often than men; they have higher levels of prescription and non-prescription drug use; they undergo more surgical procedures; in self-report studies, women report suffering from more illness and experiencing poorer health than men. Thus, although men have higher rates of some of the chronic diseases (such as cardiovascular diseases) that constitute the leading causes of death, men are actually sick less often than women.

These gender differences in mortality and morbidity raise interesting questions about why, if women are consistently favoured by lower risk of premature death, they generally experience poorer health and seek medical help more often than men. Such questions reinforce the contention that women's health merits a more prominent focus within health psychology. In fact, the apparently paradoxical gender differences in mortality and morbidity argue very strongly for a comparative approach.

Many factors could potentially contribute to the differences between men and women in mortality and morbidity. At a psychological level, it is almost certain that gender differences, in attention to and representation of symptomatology, play a part, as do differences between men and women in their willingness to report symptoms to physicians and others. At a biological level, it is probable that men and women vary in their constitutional predispositions to certain disorders. Clearly, women suffer *exclusively* from disorders related to their particular reproductive role and, while men may be more likely to develop cardiovascular disease, women are much more vulnerable to some disabling chronic diseases such as rheumatoid arthritis. In fact, the existence of health concerns that are exclusive to women (such as issues surrounding pregnancy and birth, menstrual cycle disorders, hysterectomy, breast and cervical cancer) or that disproportionately affect women (rheumatoid arthritis, eating disorders, depression) constitutes another important reason why the study of women's health deserves a higher priority.

PSYCHOLOGICAL STRESS

A key concept in health psychology is psychological stress. It is also a concept that may help make some sense of these apparently paradoxical gender differences in mortality and morbidity. Men and women may vary in the degree to which they encounter stress. They may also differ in the sorts of stresses to which they are conventionally exposed, in their appraisal of stress, in the psychological and biological impact of stress and in their characteristic coping strategies and behavior in the face of stress. As Baum and Grunberg (1991) argued, psychological stress "has been linked to differences in health and illness among different groups of people and, in particular, provides a rich array of points of interaction with gender" (p. 80). They further asserted that "differences in stress appraisal, in coping, or in one of the many forms of response or adaptation could singly or together predispose men and women to different illnesses and health problems" (p. 80).

Let us first try to indicate what we mean by the term psychological stress. In spite of its pivotal position in health psychology, it has proved surprisingly difficult to obtain agreement among researchers as to the precise meaning of psychological stress. However, given the extent to which the term is now part of everyday vocabulary and that most people have some common understanding of what it signifies, issues of precise definition need not detain us over-much.

The American physiologist, Walter Cannon (1935) was among the first to use the term stress in a non-engineering context and clearly regarded it as a disturbing force, something which upset the person's equilibrium, disrupted the usual balance. Cannon applied the term homeostasis when referring to this equilibrium or balance. From a perspective such as this, then, psychological stress refers to those events or situations that challenge a person's psychological and/or physiological homeostasis. Stressful circumstances are those which do not permit easy accommodation. Because of their meaning and the nature of the information they contain, individuals have to mobilize extensive psychological and/or physiological resources to deal with them; they cannot be handled 'on automatic'.

Stress is not, however, an objective characteristic of the environment. The point is nowhere better illustrated than in the research and writings of Richard Lazarus, Susan Folkman, and colleagues. For an event or situation to be stressful, according to Lazarus and Folkman (1984), we have to perceive or appraise it as such. Other, i.e. non-threatening appraisals would serve to diminish the disruptive impact of the event and short-circuit the stress. An experimental study reported by Lazarus *et al.* (1965) affords a good illustration here. Subjects viewed a potentially stressful film called *Woodshop*, which depicted a series of gruesome accidents at a sawmill, such as a worker severing a finger. One group of subjects were encouraged to adopt a denial appraisal, by informing them prior to viewing the film, that the participants in it were actors, that the events were staged, and that no one was really injured. A second group were encouraged to use an intellectualization appraisal and view the film from the vantage of its likely impact as a vehicle for promoting safety at work. A third group of subjects viewed the film without prior instructions. Heart rate and skin conductance were monitored throughout to gauge the physiological impact of the film and subjects were asked to rate subjective feelings of stress. Those who had received either denial or intellectualization instructions showed less physiological reaction to the film and reported that it was less stressful than subjects given no appraisal instructions.

Thus, particular appraisals can ameliorate the impact of a potentially stressful event. There is a lesson of general significance to be learnt from this demonstration; there are psychological mechanisms at our disposal which serve to combat potential stress. The existence of such devices has been recognized for some time. Freud referred to them as defense mechanisms, although today they are generally called coping strategies and, to an extent, they help explain why, in the face of a potentially stressful situation, some people become stressed but others do not. Part of the explanation is that some individuals have a fuller repertoire of psychological coping strategies. However, this is far from a complete explanation. Most current models of stress and illness, for example, postulate that stress is more likely to precipitate illness where there is an existing vulnerability, a diathesis as it is usually called.

It is possible to regard this vulnerability as operating on a number of levels. First of all, it can operate on a biological level. Some individuals may simply be predisposed to suffer disruption to specific biological systems in the face of stress, for example individuals have been found to vary markedly in their cardiovascular reactions to psychological stress. This variability, to an extent, reflects genetic predisposition; monozygotic twins show much greater concordance of reaction than dizygotic twins (see eg. Carroll *et al.*, 1985). Consider briefly the case of pepsinogen and susceptibility to ulcers. Pepsinogen secretory activity also shows a marked genetic influence (Mirsky, 1958. A classic study reported by Weiner *et al.*, (1957) indicated just how stress and biological vulnerability can interact to produce disease. The subjects were new recruits in the U.S. army. Prior to their basic training, which is generally conceded to be extremely stressful, gastrointestinal examinations were undertaken. On the basis of the results, two groups of soldiers were selected, a group of oversecretors of pepsinogen and a group of undersecretors. None of the selected soldiers had ulcers at this stage. Approximately four months later, at the end of basic training, the soldiers were re-examined. Fourteen per cent of the oversecretors had now developed ulcers, whereas none of the undersecretors had. Thus stress itself is a necessary but insufficient condition for illness; diathesis, in this case in the form of biological predisposition, must also be present.

Vulnerability may also operate at a purely psychological level. People vary in the stock of coping strategies they can tap and in their habitual coping styles. Not all of these are beneficial to health. For example, type A behaviour is a coping style where diverse environmental provocations are dealt with by competitiveness, time urgency and hostility. While some counter-evidence exists, it would appear that, for those employed in white collar occupations at least, some components of type A behavior, most notably hostility, constitute a risk factor for coronary heart disease (see, eg. Bennett and Carroll, 1990). On the other hand, repressed hostility and passivity seem to characterize ulcer patients (eg. Lyketsos *et al.*, 1982). Other coping styles are more positively indicated. Aside from type B behaviour (ie. the absence of type A characteristics) offering protection in the context of coronary heart disease, there is now evidence emerging that a coping style which involves denial is associated with a more positive prognosis following mastectomy (surgical removal of the breast performed as a treatment for cancer).

Pettingale and colleagues (1985) characterized four broad styles of coping from women's responses to interviews conducted four months after mastectomy. These were 'stoic acceptance', 'denial', 'fighting spirit', and 'helplessness/hopelessness'. Examination five years after the operation indicated that coping style was related to recurrence-free survival. Women who adopted either the 'denial' or 'fighting spirit' approaches fared much better. In addition, Pettingale *et al.* (1981) found that immune functioning, as indexed by immunoglobulin levels, was better in women using denial to cope than in those relying on the other strategies. In a more recent study, Dean and Surtees (1989) again interviewed women with breast cancer three months after mastectomy, and allocated them, on the basis of their interview responses, to one of the four previously mentioned coping styles. Outcome was examined in terms of the approach the women indicated they had adopted. Only 'denial' emerged from the analysis as offering an advantage in terms of disease recurrence or mortality.

The use of more specific coping strategies, such as those associated with physical and mental relaxation, has also been shown to be related to a more positive outcome, as for instance when individuals are faced with surgery (Kaplan *et al.*, 1982) or cancer treatment (Burish and Redd, 1983), or experiencing childbirth (Niven, 1992), or suffering from chronic pain (Malone and Strube, 1988).

Individuals may also be rendered vulnerable at a social level. What might be broadly termed social support appears to serve as a buffer countering the worst ravages of stress. By social support is meant the provision of comfort, caring, esteem, or help by other people or social groups. There is a growing body of evidence that social support offers protective advantage in a number of areas of health and well-being: pregnancy (Oakley, 1988); labor pain (Niven, 1985); childbirth (Klaus *et al.*, 1986); breast feeding (Lewis, 1986); post-natal adjustment (Elliot *et al.*, 1988); parenting of a child with Down's Syndrome (Sloper *et al.*, 1991); depression (Brown and Harris, 1978); coronary heart disease (Orth-Gomér and Unden, 1990); recovery from a major coronary event (Fontana *et al.*, 1989); atherosclerosis (Blumenthal *et al.*, 1987); cancer (Scherg and Blohmke, 1988). This is a matter to which we shall return in the final chapter.

In a parallel fashion, stress itself can be regarded as eliciting effects at a number of levels. As Steptoe (1984) indicated, there are at least three basic routes through which stress can contribute to ill-health. First of all, stress can disrupt physiological homeostasis, provoking marked reactions in various biological systems. A substantial body of research testifies that a range of both laboratory and everyday challenges are highly provocative to the cardiovascular system (see eg. Krantz and Manuck, 1984). Further, there is also evidence that the magnitude of such effects are related to cardiovascular disease risk status. For example, young persons who are at risk of hypertension by virtue of elevated, although sub-hypertensive, resting blood pressure levels show more pronounced reactions to stress than low-risk normotensive subjects (see eg. Carroll *et al.*, 1991).

There is also a vast catalog of research which indicates that psychological stress elicits marked neuroendocrine responses, particularly increased catecholamine activity (Frankenhaeuser, 1983). Given that adrenalin has a powerful lipid mobilizing effect, it is perhaps no surprise to find that psychological stress is also associated with increases in cholesterol level. For example, van Doornen and van Blokland (1987) monitored the serum cholesterol levels of students on a normal, routine day and on the day of an examination. Cholesterol levels were significantly higher on the day of the examination.

Finally, evidence is accumulating that psychological stress compromises the efficiency of the immune system. Examinations (Kiecolt-Glaser *et al.*, 1986), marital status and marital disruption (Kiecolt-Glaser *et al.*, 1987), and unemployment (Arnetz *et al.*, 1987) have all been revealed to have deleterious effects.

Stress can also exert an influence at a behavioral level. Certain behaviors, cigarette smoking, excessive alcohol consumption, particular dietary habits, low levels of physical activity and exercise, have all been identified as contributing negatively to physical health and as positive risk factors for a range of diseases. While such behaviors have complex determinants, it is likely that one determinant is psychological stress. There is evidence that the incidence of such unhealthy behaviors increases during periods of stress. Consider the example of smoking. In two similar experiments, Schachter and his colleagues (see eg. Schachter, 1978) manipulated psychological stress while ostensibly measuring tactile sensitivity. In the high stress condition, such sensitivity was measured by the administration, sporadically over the session, of a series of intense, fairly painful electric shocks. In the low stress condition, the shocks were almost imperceptible. Between testing periods, the subjects, who were all smokers, were free to smoke or not as they wished. In both studies, subjects smoked considerably more in high than in low stress conditions. Another example emanates from a 'real world' study by Farrant (1980) who found that women awaiting the results of pre-natal tests for fetal abnormality were more likely to smoke during this period.

Finally, stress may influence subjective symptomatology and what is called illness behavior. Individuals vary markedly in the extent to which they perceive, acknowledge and respond to physical symptoms. At one end of the scale we have hypochondriasis, where individuals are pathologically obsessed by symptomatology and constantly behave as if seriously ill, and at the other end, instances of sudden death, where there was little or no previously acknowledged symptomatology or medical consultation.

It is possible that psychological stress may be one factor prompting individuals to attend more to symptoms of illness and seek medical advice. House and colleagues (1979) have presented an example. Subjective complaints of skin rashes and upper respiratory difficulties, coughs and excessive sputum, in a group of industrial workers were compared with reports of stress at work. Work stress was not reliably associated with actual medical evidence of dermatological or respiratory problems. However those who reported most stress at work, complained most of physical symptoms. Thus the relationship between stress at work and apparent respiratory and dermatological disorders held only for subjective complaints of such disorders.

GENDER AND STRESS

As indicated, people vary in their vulnerability to stress. Some of these vulnerability variations exist at a biological level. There is also substantial evidence that acute psychological stressors disrupt a number of biological systems. It is possible that the extent and patterns of disruption differ between men and women. In a subsequent chapter, Light and Girdler explore such differences in cardiovascular reactions to stress. It is sufficient at the moment to record that there is emerging evidence that women display a tendency toward greater heart rate increases during stress compared to men; men, on the other hand, show higher systolic blood pressure reactions.

There would also appear to be differences in neuroendocrine reactions to stress. Conventionally, women show less marked reactions (see eg. van Doornen, 1986). However, such gender differences in physiological response may interact with behavioral orientation. For example, Collins and Frankenhauser (1978) observed that female students studying engineering in technical school tended to exhibit neuro-endocrine stress reactions more typical of males. These data were interpreted as reflecting a more masculine orientation toward achievement demands in these female engineering students. In broad terms then, as Matthews *et al.* (1991) pointed out, it is possible that gender differences in biological reactions to psychological stress reflect differences in the way women and men conventionally cope with demands in traditional male areas of competency. Presumably, such variations would dissipate or even be reversed when women and men are required to cope with challenges in areas of traditional female competency. Lundberg *et al.* (1981) compared neuroendocrine stress reactions in mothers and fathers accompanying their three year old children to hospital for a check-up. They suggested that this demanding but non-competitive situation dealing with the traditional female concerns for their children would tap an area of female rather than male competency. While there were no gender differences in secretion of adrenaline and cortisol in this situation, the mothers showed greater non-adrenaline reactivity than the fathers, suggesting that the usual reaction of women to stress can be altered if the stressor taps a female domain of competence.

We are also without evidence of whether women and men differ in terms of the impact of stress on their immune systems. Given that there appear to be consistent gender differences in unstressed immune function, eg. women appear to display larger antibody responses to a variety of antigens and, at the same time, show weaker cell-mediated immune reactions (see Baum and Grunberg, 1991) and that women exhibit increased susceptibility to a variety of auto-immune disorders, such as multiple schlerosis or rheumatoid arthritis, the exploration of gender, stress, and immune function could prove fruitful.

As indicated previously, individuals might be vulnerable at a psychological or behavioral level, and stress can affect the incidence of unhealthy behavior. It is possible that women differ from men in the ways in whcih they conventionally cope with stress, ie. perhaps men cope with stress in a manner which renders them particularly susceptible to major, life-threatening disorders such as coronary heart disease and lung cancer, whereas women's experience of stress and the means by which they deal with it makes them ill more often, but less seriously. Hart (1989) has argued that men deal with stress through the use of alcohol and cigarettes; for women, stress appears pathological, and as a consequence they have resorted to medical advice which is reflected in much higher rates of diagnoses of depressive illness and recorded tranquilliser use. In other words, Hart concluded, female stress has been medicalized and women have become the clients of doctors, the passive consumers of medical rather than market drugs. Indeed, it has been estimated that around half the difference between male and female death rates can be accounted for by differences in cigarette and alcohol consumption (Waldron, 1976). However, this situation may be changing since recent figures show that smoking rates in women continue to increase, while those in men decrease (Waldron, in press), and that so-called 'problem drinking' as well as overall alcohol consumption has increased in women (Wilsnack *et al*, 1984).

Furthermore, it is unlikely that such a straightforward explanation is sufficient. For example, in the case of coronary heart disease, taking into account traditional risk factors including cigarette smoking still leaves a gender mortality ratio of over 2 in women's favour (Wingard *et al*., 1983). The impact of behavioral factors such as smoking would also seem to interact with social and material circumstances. It is clear from research in various Western countries that social and material circumstances exert a powerful influence on mortality and morbidity and, while some have attempted to re-duce such influences to matters of individual behavior and life-style (eg. Matthews, 1989), they continue to defy easy reduction. For example, in a study conducted by Marmot and colleagues (1984) among British civil servants, mortality over a 10-year period was found to be three times greater in the lowest employment grades relative to the highest grades. Further, the greatest part of this difference could not be explained by recourse to smoking, cholesterol levels and reported physical activity. On the basis of an extensive survey of health and lifestyle, Blaxter (1990) concluded that, for the bulk of the population, behavior is rarely totally healthy or totally unhealthy and that, for this great majority, health is primarily affected by the social and material environment.

She went on to assert that "It is among those who are not environmentally vulnerable that harmful behavioral habits such as smoking appear to produce a greater effect" (Blaxter, 1990, p. 231). Thus, behavioral factors would appear to exert a considerably stronger influence on the health of those in the best material circumstances; yet it is among those in the most meagre circumstances that health is poorest and mortality rates highest.

This raises a general issue concerning the influence of social and material circumstances on women's health and on gender differences. The available data suggest that social status affects women's mortality and morbidity in much the same way as men's. However, issues emerge regarding the manner in which women's social status is characterized. Traditionally, epidemiologists have classified women on the basis of the occupation of the head of the household, usually defined as the husband in married couples. More recently, researchers (see eg. Arber, 1989) have argued that this is inappropriate and that, anyway, material, asset-based measures, such as housing tenure and car-ownership, constitute more proper indices of social and material circumstances than occupation-based classification systems. Using such asset-based measures Arber found that health differentials for women are as large as those for men. However, whether occupation-based or asset-based measures are adopted, adverse health among women is concentrated among those whose material circumstances and employment position are least favourable. Lack of employment outside the home emerges as a correlate of poor health for women, as well as men (see eg. Cochrane, 1983) and of course more women than men are not employed outside the home. For British women, aged 15–59, house ownership status, coupled with family car ownership, reduced their standardized mortality ratio to almost half the recorded for women who possessed neither of these material assets (Moser and Goldblatt, 1985), while lack of a car has been found to be associated with significantly higher levels of psychosomatic symptomology indicative of stress in mothers of handicapped children (Sloper *et al.*, 1991).

As the reader will recall, it has been argued that women differ from men in how they judge their own health and in their consequent health-reporting behavior. As we have seen, there is evidence that stress can influence subjective symptomatology, disclosure and general illness behavior. Many authors (see eg. Hart, 1989) have suggested that this is a particular feature of female coping styles. It would certainly appear to be the case that women are more likely than men to report symptoms, more likely to seek medical attention and more likely to use health service care and provision (Mechanic, 1982).

There are a number of possible reasons for this. Experiences such as menstruation, pregnancy and childbirth cause women to focus more on bodily sensations than men. These experiences bring them into more frequent contact with health care professionals and this contact continues throughout the early years of parenting, thus encouraging the recorded reporting of symptoms and the use of health care provisions. Furthermore, Miles (1991) has suggested that conventionally appropriate behavior for women includes far more personal disclosure than is the case for men and that structural differences in the lives of women (work, life style, etc.) are likely to have a bearing. Additionally, substantial cultural messages encourage the view that health is women's preserve. Even when these messages, as is frequently the case, are targetted at the health concerns of men and of children, it is women who are urged to take the responsibility. Thus, advertisements cajole women to switch to low fat margarine instead of butter to preserve their husbands' hearts (Karpf, 1988). Finally, according to

Miles, the concept of female frailty has wide social currency. It has certainly been reinforced by the medical profession. As Ehrenreich and English (1979) pointed out, medical practice in the latter part of last century and the beginning of this has very much been guided by the view that it was women's normal state to be ill. However, it remains unclear as to what extent gender differences in symptom registration and reporting account for differences in experienced morbidity as opposed to recorded morbidity. It should also be noted as Rodin and Ickovics (1990) have indicated that not all research points to substantial gender variation in illness behavior.

As implied in the previous discussion, gender differences in the biological impact of stress and the psychological mechanisms that are conventionally adopted to cope with stress undoubtedly contribute to women and men's differing health profiles. However, such considerations are unlikely to afford a complete explanation. The precise pattern of challenges and stresses that men and women face is also likely to be of significance. Gender differences in social role and role expectation are likely to color not only how women and men deal with stress, but the precise environmental stresses that they are exposed to, for example those involved in parenting which continues to be predominantly a female concern and those which they appraise to be stressful. If this is the case, one would expect that, as social expectations and broad environmental circumstances of women and men converge, so too would indices of health. There is evidence to support this. For example, Leviatan and Cohen (1985) found that the life expectancy gender gap was much less for men and women living in a kibbutz than the figure conventionally recorded. At birth, the gap was 4.5 years in the kibbutz in contrast to the 7.1 years that emerges from comparable international data; at age 50 years the respective figures were 2.7 and 5.1 years. This narrowing of the gender gap reflected improvements in male life expectancy rather than reductions in female life expectancy. Unfortunately, other evidence of convergence depends upon a declining advantage for women who are now more susceptible to death from heart disease and to cancer, relative to men, than they were in the past (Strickland, 1988).

Finally, as noted earlier, people may be rendered vulnerable to stress at a social level, ie. have few positive social resources at their disposal. We have already discussed emerging evidence that occupational and material status are important factors in health. Related to such matters is the broad concept of social support. Few social scientists would now question the proposition that low levels of social support are associated with poor physical and mental health. Unfortunately, as Shumaker and Hill (1991) pointed out, much of the research into social support and health, particularly physical health, has focussed on men. In contrast, the issue of social support and women's health has been relatively neglected, except perhaps in the area of reproductive health. It is possible that gender differences in the extent and nature of social support provision might contribute to gender health variations. Alternatively, women may differ from men in terms of the health consequences of social support. These are matters to which we shall return in the final chapter. It is sufficient here to note that considerations concerning social support are likely to be of substantial importance.

CONCLUSION

In this chapter we have sought to explore some of the issues surrounding gender and health and the apparent paradox that, while men die earlier than women, women suffer from more illness. While the gender mortality gap generally gives women an advantage of between 6 and 7 years of life, well-life expectancy, a measure which adjusts standard life expectancy for health-related quality of life, leaves women and men much closer. Kaplan, Anderson and Wingard (1991) estimated that, for American men, the well-life expectancy was 60 whereas for women it was 63 years.

Our current focus has been on stress and its biological and psychological impact. Evidence is accumulating that women and men may vary in their exposure to and appraisal of psychological stress (women certainly report experiencing more stress), their patterns of biological reaction to stress, and the coping mechanisms that are conventionally deployed. However, we are still far from a satisfactory account of how such differences contribute to gender variations in health profile. What is clear is that the relationships between health on the one hand and psychological and social factors on the other are exceedingly complex and that gender considerations increase this complexity. Nevertheless, satisfactory solutions are not well served by scientific attention being overly preoccupied with the health of men. Robust models within health psychology are much more likely to emerge from a fuller consideration of women's health and the adoption of a genuinely comparative approach. As Baum and Grunberg (1991) so cogently argued, "Research on health and behaviour should consider men *and* women – not because it is discrimatory not to do so – but because it is good science" (Baum and Grunberg, 1991, p. 84). This, such an approach should ultimately benefit both men and women. It could also be argued that health psychology research might more usefully focus on women since women are the survivors and the carers of parents, partners, friends and children. Therefore, their health is crucial to the health of the entire population.

Finally, health psychologists must also appreciate that other sociodemographic factors, most notably social and material circumstances and ethnicity, undeniably cut across and almost certainly interact with the influences of gender. We firmly believe that an increased attention to interactive influences of this sort would markedly benefit our understanding of the social, psychological, and psycho-biological processes of illness and disease, and provide more informed guidance in matters of treatment, prevention, and health promotion.

FURTHER READING

Baum, A. and Grunberg, N.E. (1991). Gender, stress, and health. *Health Psychology*, 10, 80–85.
Miles, (1991). *Women, health and medicine*. Milton Keynes: Open University Press.
Rodin, J. and Ickovics, J.R. (1990). Women's health: Review and research agenda as we approach the 21st century. *American Psychologist*, 45, 1018–1034.

2

WOMEN, MOOD AND THE MENSTRUAL CYCLE

CYNTHIA GRAHAM AND JOHN BANCROFT

MRC Reproductive Biology Unit (Behavioural Research Group), Kennedy Tower, Royal Edinburgh Hospital, Morningside Park, Edinburgh EH10 5HF, Scotland, UK

However much we may argue about the degree and importance of gender differences, particularly those of a cognitive or behavioral kind, the essential differences between men and women lie within their reproductive biology. Whether a woman experiences pregnancy or not, she will menstruate. Modern woman spends a much smaller proportion of her reproductive span pregnant or lactating and hence menstruates far more often than her forbears. Menstruation is a recurrent reminder of her reproductive femaleness.

The human menstrual cycle is a complex process involving interaction between the hypothalamus, pituitary gland and ovary. By convention, the first day of menstrual bleeding is regarded as the start of the cycle. This is followed by a gradual rise in pituitary gonadotrophic hormones, follicle stimulating hormone (FSH) and luteinising hormone (LH). These stimulate the developing follicle of the ovary which, in turn, secretes steroid hormones, in particular estradiol. As the estradiol level rises, it eventually triggers a surge of LH which, in turn, provokes the release of the ovum from the follicle. The burst follicle then transforms into a corpus luteum which proceeds to produce both estradiol and progesterone; these together act on the endometrium of the uterus to prepare it for the possible implantation of a fertilized ovum. If this does not occur, the levels of both hormones fall, menstrual bleeding occurs and the cycle starts all over again. The provocation of the LH surge by the rising level of estradiol, or 'positive feedback', is one of the clearest functional characteristics that distinguishes the brains of women and men. Apart from the essential rise and fall in levels of ovarian hormones, cyclical variations are occurring in a wide variety of physiological systems, including the immune system, the capillaries of muscle, skin and other tissues as well as the endometrial lining of the uterus. Many of these changes are ill-understood (Asso, 1983).

MENSTRUAL CYCLE-RELATED CHANGES

Negative views of menstruation are longstanding. In many societies, particularly preindustrial, it has been endowed with mystic significance, often the subject of taboo. The menstruating woman is seen as 'unclean', a source of pollution, or a threat of some kind and is often barred from religious ceremonies (Shuttle and Redgrove, 1986).

Reflecting this negative symbolism, the traditional view is that menstruation is a predominantly negative experience for women, involving unpleasant physical changes such as pain, bloating or tender breasts, or negative moods such as irritability or depression. It is important to remember, however, that for many women, menstruation is free from unpleasant symptoms and is a reassuring reminder of their 'normality' or, in those seeking to avoid pregnancy, their non-pregnant state.

Furthermore, although a proportion of women do report cyclical changes in their mood and physical state, such changes involve 'good' as well as 'bad' phases. It is noteworthy that little attention has been paid to these positive changes related to the menstrual cycle. The emphasis is usually on a negative pattern of low mood, low energy and irritability occurring premenstrually and/or during menstruation. As we shall see below, research to date in this area has been plagued by methodological problems and the proportion of women who experience cyclical changes in mood, either positive or negative, as well as the etiology of such changes, is unknown.

Although the nature and significance of menstrual cycle-related changes in mood remains unclear, this subject is of importance for a number of reasons. Firstly, whatever the cause, some women do regard cyclical mood change as a significant problem which interferes with their social or occupational functioning. Secondly, it is possible that the propensity for such cyclical changes is linked in some way with the tendency for some women to react adversely to oral contraceptives, or to hormonal changes associated with pregnancy and the menopause. The possibility that cyclical mood change is a precursor, or a trigger, for depressive illness (estimated to be twice as common in women than in men, particularly women in their reproductive years) has also been raised.

Finally, there are important political implications surrounding this issue. In recent years, there has been an increased awareness and interest in women's health issues and, at the same time, a medicalization of women's 'problems'. Menstrual cycle-related mood changes have increasingly been defined as a medical problem, the 'premenstrual syndrome' and one for which medical treatment is appropriate, despite the lack of agreement about why the syndrome occurs or what is effective intervention.

This process of medicalization can be seen as having both positive and negative consequences. On the one hand, women's experiences of menstruation and menopause, previously ignored by the medical profession, have become the subject of serious research attention. On the other hand, medicalization encourages the idea that women experiencing cyclical mood changes are in some way 'ill', which serves to undermine their sense of self-sufficiency and self-esteem.

The role of premenstrual symptoms in criminal behavior has also become of interest, with a number of legal cases where premenstrual syndrome has been accepted as a mitigating factor in manslaughter, arson and assault (Boorse, 1987). Further controversy has arisen with the proposal that premenstrual mood changes be established as a diagnostic category in the Diagnostic and Statistical Manual of Mental Disorders (DSM III-R) as 'Late Luteal Phase Dysphoric Disorder'.

For these various reasons, it is not surprising that the menstrual cycle and its impact on the well-being of women remains a highly contentious issue. It has become something of a battleground for those who contest the relative importance of biological and social determinants of gender role differences. As part of the polemic, those who regard women as unsuitable for positions of greater social responsibility often focus on the menstrual cycle as the basis of their biological vulnerability; those who view women as fit as, or fitter than, men may minimize the significance of the menstrual cycle, and attribute any disadvantages associated with it to the negative effects of social learning. The controversy has therefore centered on the question of whether cyclical variations in mood are a function of the biological processes involved in the menstrual cycle or rather a consequence of social learning, expectation and attribution.

Presenting a dispassionate account of the relevance of the menstrual cycle to the well-being of women is consequently not easy. It will readily fall prey to the accusation that, from one point of view it is too biological and from the other, too sociological. In this chapter we will consider the extent to which women experience variations in their well-being and mood that are predictably linked to the menstrual cycle and the relative importance of psychosocial and biological factors in accounting for such variations. We will not attempt to present an exhaustive review of the literature but, instead, highlight some of the many unresolved issues in this area and then suggest an alternative explanatory model which incorporates biological, psychological and sociological influences on women's experience of their menstrual cycles.

THE PREMENSTRUAL SYNDROME

Dominating the above debate is the concept of 'the premenstrual syndrome' (PMS). This vague and ill-defined concept contains the notion that there is a pathological state affecting many women which is manifested as unpleasant mood and physical symptoms typically occurring during the premenstrual part of the menstrual cycle, remitting at or soon after the onset of menstrual bleeding.

PMS is an unsatisfactory concept for many reasons. It fails to make any distinction between a cyclical variation in well-being and physical state which many women may experience but do not regard as a significant problem (and which presumably is in some sense a normal phenomenon) and distressing changes in mood and behavior, which can have significant effects on a woman's life. The reason why the concept is highly contentious is therefore obvious. If it is believed that the recurrent tendency to marked mood and behavioral changes shown by a small proportion of women is the more extreme version of cyclical mood change associated with the normal menstrual cycle of all women, then the view that women are incapacitated by their menstrual cycles, showing erratic and uncontrollable behavior at 'that time of the month', appears strengthened. If, on the other hand, such phenomena can be attributed to the effects of negative social conditioning and are basically independent of biological processes, then premenstrual 'symptoms' are seen as further evidence of the repressed position of women in our society and of the use of menstruation as a justification for restricting women's roles.

Thus, we have the contrasting evidence of those doctors who recommend drastic surgical or medical procedures for the treatment of severe PMS, such as hysterectomy and oöphorectomy (surgical removal of the uterus and ovaries) or the use of powerful hormonal regimens such as LHRH (lutenizing hormone releasing hormone) agonists, and of those social scientists whose experiments purport to show that premenstrual symptoms are the result of expectation and attribution. Let us, therefore, examine the concept of PMS in more detail.

Definition

The lack of an agreed-upon operational definition of PMS has contributed to the inconclusive and conflicting research findings. Disagreement has mainly centered on the following issues:

1. The symptoms experienced and their temporal pattern in relation to the menstrual cycle.
2. The severity of symptoms required for a diagnosis of PMS.
3. The baseline against which premenstrual changes should be measured.
4. Whether the symptoms constitute one syndrome or several.

The changes which have been associated with PMS are extremely diverse and, as a result of this, there has been general agreement that it is the timing, rather than the type of symptoms which should determine whether a woman suffers from the syndrome. However, there have been a number of different temporal patterns described. Some women report a dramatic alleviation of their premenstrual symptoms with the onset of menstrual bleeding but for others the symptoms, while starting during the premenstrual phase, may be as severe, or even at their peak, during the menstrual period. Researchers have tended to focus more on 'premenstrual' changes, often ignoring the menstrual phase altogether. It is possible that different mechanisms are involved in these different temporal patterns.

Dalton (1984), one of the principal proponents of the concept of PMS, defined it as "the recurrence of symptoms in the premenstruum with absence of symptoms in the postmenstruum" (p. 3). Not only does this definition fail to specify the severity of symptoms required, but the stipulation that there be a complete *absence* of symptoms in the postmenstrual period is problematic. As the symptoms reported premenstrually are not specific to PMS, this requirement would preclude the possibility of any physical or emotional symptom occurring at any other time of the cycle! Recognizing this difficulty, Halbreich and Endicott (1985) suggested that there be a significant *change* in symptoms premenstrually from some specified 'baseline', although the question of the appropriate baseline, against which premenstrual change should be measured, remains.

The consistency of premenstrual changes is also an issue. Some operational definitions require an arbitrary criterion of cyclicity to be met consistently over several consecutive cycles yet there is evidence that most women showed marked inter-cycle variability in premenstrual changes (Hart *et al.* 1987). Both in terms of timing and consistency, conventional definitions exclude large proportions of women from the category of PMS on arbitrary grounds, when there is no logical reason to assume that they are etiologically distinct. Thus, we see an example of 'medical constructionism': an entity which persists as a result of a self-reinforcing definition and is used to account for a wide range of problems but which, as rigidly defined, applies to only a small proportion of women.

This constructionism has had an adverse effect on research; many studies have excluded those cases which do not fit some arbitrary definition of 'PMS'. An example of this are the diagnostic criteria developed by Haskett *et al.* (1980), who argued for a single, "primary recurrent premenstrual tension syndrome". Their criteria include the requirements that there be: (1) at least five different types of mood and behavioral symptoms; (2) appearance of symptoms only during the premenstrual phase, with relief soon after menses; (3) symptoms present for at least six consecutive cycles.

Definitions based on the timing, rather than the type of symptoms have resulted in 'PMS' covering a variety of phenomena with probably heterogeneous etiologies. There is as yet no good reason to assume, for example, that cyclical breast tenderness has the same biological basis as cyclical depression, beyond their tendency to co-vary with the ovarian cycle. Studies which have compared women using and not using oral contraceptives have found that the two groups can be differentiated on the basis of premenstrual physical symptoms, such as breast tenderness, but are very similar in patterns of cyclical mood change (Walker and Bancroft, 1990; Graham and Sherwin, 1992), suggesting that the physical and psychological symptoms may have different determinants.

Assessment

One of the most frequent criticisms of studies on PMS has been their reliance on retrospective self-reports of symptoms. Retrospective methods ask women either whether they *usually* experience cyclical changes or have done so during their most recent menstrual cycle(s), whereas prospective methods require women to rate their subjective state, usually on a daily basis. There is now considerable evidence that these two methods do not correlate well. It has been argued that women over-estimate the symptoms experienced or report their 'worst experience' on retrospective ratings. This has led to a tendency to reject any form of retrospective assessment and to recommend daily prospective ratings, in a fairly uncritical manner, as the only acceptable method of documenting PMS. However, the use of daily ratings is not without its own problems. This relatively demanding procedure leads to low compliance and the introduction of other sources of bias. The process of daily ratings may well influence the woman's current experience, particularly with changes that have a natural tendency to vary in intensity from month to month in any case. Most criteria of cyclicity based on daily ratings use average scores of a defined period, eg. the premenstrual week. Most women do not assess their past experiences in terms of average ratings in this way but are more likely to evaluate a specific time period, such as the premenstrual week in terms of its 'worst days'.

There are other possible explanations for the discrepancy found between retrospective and prospective reports. The procedure used to evaluate the two types of assessment has typically involved comparing a woman's retrospective rating of one or two premenstrual symptoms (ie. her 'usual' experience) with her prospective score on these items during one cycle. However, because of the considerable variation in severity between cycles, the daily ratings from one cycle may not be representative of a woman's usual experience (Hart *et al.*, 1987). Moreover, the criterion that women show a significant degree of change on one or two specific symptoms may also be overly stringent if the precise changes women experience vary from cycle to cycle.

For many research purposes, eg. prevalence studies, the low compliance associated with prospective methods is a serious handicap. Retrospective questionnaires can prove useful both as initial screening instruments and for use in studying the relationships between symptom reporting and other variables. There is, therefore, a need to develop more satisfactory retrospective methods of assessment.

Prevalence

The lack of an accepted definition of PMS and other methodological problems has precluded any valid estimates of the prevalence of this condition. Moreover, many prevalence studies have not attempted to quantify the severity of symptoms experienced, resulting in prevalence estimates which vary widely, from 25 per cent to almost 100 per cent (Andersch et al., 1986). Awareness of premenstrual physical changes, such as breast tenderness or bloating, are reported by a substantial majority of women and could be regarded as normal physiological changes. Mood changes are reported less frequently; irritability is probably the most common, though usually of mild degree. When severity of changes is assessed, there is some consensus across studies that between 2 and 10 percent of women are experiencing changes which they find problematic (Logue and Moos, 1986).

A number of 'risk factors', ie. variables which increase an individual's vulnerability to premenstrual change, have been studied, but here too there are few consistent findings. For example, although it is often asserted that PMS is more common in older women, a number of studies have found no correlation between age and the reporting of PMS (Logue and Moos, 1986). On the other hand, a consistent observation has been that women attending PMS clinics or volunteering for treatment studies tend to be in their thirties (Freeman et al., 1985; Bancroft et al., 1992).

Etiological Theories – Biological

An extensive body of research exists in which biological determinants of PMS have been sought. Until very recently, this research has been guided by the basic assumption that women who suffer from premenstrual symptoms do so as a consequence of some abnormality of their ovarian or menstrual cycle. Etiological theories have postulated a relative deficiency of progesterone, a relative excess of estradiol, deficiencies of vitamins or trace elements, an excess of stress-related hormones such as prolactin or cortisol, among many other biological explanations. The usual paradigm has been to measure 'factor X' at various points during the second half of the menstrual cycle (often at only one or two points) in women who have been categorized as either 'PMS sufferers' or 'non-sufferers'. No replicable abnormality has been demonstrated in this way (Bancroft and Backstrom, 1985; Rubinow et al., 1988). With the wisdom of hindsight, we should perhaps express little surprise at this overwhelming body of negative results. The menstrual cycle is a highly complex and dynamic process, with a veritable cascade of interacting and self-regulating mechanisms. It is, therefore, little wonder that arbitrary periodic sampling of this system to measure one factor or another has proved fruitless. Most researchers now agree that there is no simple hormonal deficiency or excess associated with premenstrual changes; indeed, as we shall discuss below, the relevant factor that distinguishes the PMS sufferer from the non-sufferer may not even lie in her ovarian cycle.

Etiological theories – Psychosocial

A number of investigators (eg. Ruble, 1977) have proposed that women's reports of premenstrual symptomatology may reflect social expectancies and stereotypical beliefs about the changes associated with the menstrual cycle rather than their actual experience of such symptoms. Experiments have shown that a woman's report of premenstrual symptoms can be manipulated by altering her beliefs about menstrual cycle-related changes or her expectation of when she is going to menstruate (Ruble, 1977). Evidence from other studies suggests that symptom reports are exaggerated when subjects are aware of the menstrual cycle 'focus' of a study (Parlee, 1982), although this is not a consistent finding (eg. Van den Akker and Steptoe, 1985). Finally, there is research showing that there are shared, cultural beliefs about the effects of the menstrual cycle on women's psychological and physical state (Parlee, 1982).

Results from the above studies have been used to support the notion that premenstrual symptoms are the result of expectation and attribution; the expectation that one feels worse in the premenstrual phase of the cycle because one has been taught to expect that and the attribution of negative mood states to the menstrual cycle because they happen to occur in the latter half of the cycle, whereas negative moods at other times are attributed to different factors. The onset of menstrual bleeding and the preceding physical changes are salient 'cues' and it is argued that these, combined with the shared negative beliefs about the discomfort experienced around menstruation, may lead to a distorted view of when symptoms are experienced.

Such evidence has so far been of limited relevance for two principal reasons. First, none of these studies of expectation and attribution have been carried out in women who have previously identified themselves as PMS sufferers. Subjects have predominantly been young women, often university students, the age group in which complaints of PMS are less common. It is, therefore, perfectly possible that the samples included in these studies are relatively free of such cyclical experiences. Secondly, the concealment of the researcher's interest in the menstrual cycle, whilst desirable in many respects, can be misleading. It is not unusual for women, when asked to report their subjective state, to omit to mention changes which they attribute to some factor assumed to be irrelevant. Thus, a woman who believes that an enquiry has nothing to do with her menstrual cycle may fail to mention changes which she attributes to her cycle. Conversely, a woman answering questions about her menstrual cycle may omit to mention emotional reactions which she clearly attributes to some other cause.

It is hardly surprising that studies which have involved samples of women who are not *reporting* premenstrual change have failed to demonstrate any significant cyclical variation in mood or well-being through the menstrual cycle, particularly when the menstrual cycle 'focus' is concealed. Yet these studies are often cited as evidence that PMS does not exist other than as an incorrect attribution of blame for current emotional problems on the menstrual cycle. They can only justifiably be used as evidence that symptom reports are *influenced* by expectation, shared cultural beliefs, etc. It is commonplace in clinical practice to help women to recognize the importance of other factors in their lives which may be contributing to their current distress and, as we shall see later, possibly aggravating their cyclical pattern. However, it is a cynical rejection of women's own observations and judgements, often made over many years, to account for their recurrent experience of disabling menstrual cycle-related symptoms as the simple consequence of incorrect attribution.

Treatment Approaches

The evidence of the effectiveness of medical treatment for PMS is a further powerful reflection of the ignorance and confusion that has prevailed in this research area. An extensive array of medical treatments, reflecting the bewildering number of etiological theories, have been tried. Proponents for some of these treatment approaches have made enthusiastic claims for their use (eg. Dalton, 1984), usually on the basis of clinical observation or uncontrolled studies. When placebo-controlled trials of these treatments have been carried out, they have generally failed to show any significant beneficial effect of the active treatment over placebo. The most convincing therapeutic effects have involved treatments which aim to suppress or eliminate the ovarian cycle altogether, such as LHRH agonists or the antigonadotrophic agent danazol (Sarno *et al.*, 1987), but these are in many respects drastic and associated with substantial risks of long-term use.

Perhaps the most consistent finding in treatment studies has been the high rate of 'placebo response' and in most trials, premenstrual mood changes have been more responsive to placebo than the physical symptoms (Metcalf and Hudson, 1985; Graham and Sherwin, 1992). These findings are all too readily used by some to support the idea that premenstrual mood changes are due to psychological factors such as expectation, etc. In fact there has been very little study of the 'placebo response' in its own right, although a greater understanding of its mechanism could help us to understand the underlying phenomena.

Most authors assume that beneficial effects associated with placebo are due to the administration of the placebo 'treatment' or to so-called 'non-specific' effects of the treatment regime, eg. reassurance, contact with the researcher, etc. Another possibility is that the daily monitoring of symptoms required of subjects in most studies might itself have a therapeutic effect (Endicott and Halbreich, 1982). It has also been suggested that a large component of the 'placebo response' might reflect spontaneous improvement. The month-to-month variability in symptoms has already been discussed; women entering treatment studies are likely to have been experiencing a phase of particularly severe mood change which has led them to seek treatment at this time. By the time they enter a controlled treatment study, this difficult phase may have passed its peak and they may be showing some spontaneous improvement (Bancroft and Backstrom, 1985).

One important and, in many respects, welcome consequence of the disillusionment with medical treatments has been an increasing tendency for women to seek out non-medical methods of management e.g., exercise, dietary changes, self-help groups. As yet there has been little evaluation of such approaches. Recently, methods based on 'cognitive therapy' have also been tried with some encouraging results (Morse and Dennerstein, 1988).

A RE-APPRAISAL

In a recent study (Bancroft *et al.*, 1992), women attending a gynaecology outpatient department for three different complaints – PMS, menorrhagia (excessive blood loss) and dysmenorrhoea (menstrual pain) – were compared with a control group recruited from general practice. It was found that there was considerable overlap between the three patient groups: between 55 and 69 per cent of the menorrhagic and dysmenorrhoeic group respectively regarded themselves as PMS sufferers, compared with a third of the controls. The results suggested that the presence of menstrual problems (eg. heavy bleeding or pain) aggravated any tendency to PMS with, in particular, mood changes being more severe both premenstrually and menstrually. This emphasizes the importance of considering the contribution of menstruation itself to women's experience of PMS.

In addition, a strong association was found between the experience of perimenstrual mood changes and neuroticism (N), as measured by the Eysenck Personality Inventory. Women suffering perimenstrual mood changes in each of the four groups had higher N scores than those who did not. The association between neuroticism and PMS has been demonstrated in a number of previous studies, which have also shown that the N score does not vary during the cycle and is therefore probably measuring a personality 'trait' rather than reflecting the mood 'state' associated with PMS (Mira *et al.*, 1985).

The results from this clinic study led us to postulate a 'three factor' model for understanding so-called PMS, particularly the variety that is presented in a clinical setting. These three factors are:

1. A cyclical or 'timing' factor. This assumes that the ovarian cycle, in a way not yet understood, acts as a 'biological clock' to impose or entrain a cyclical pattern on the woman's central nervous system, resulting in mood change or altered responsiveness to external events, and on peripheral tissues, resulting in cyclical changes such as breast tenderness.
2. A 'menstruation' factor, related to the processes involved in the build-up of the endometrium and its shedding during menstrual flow. The physiological changes involved in these processes clearly start well before menstruation itself and involve increasing levels of prostaglandins which we now know contribute to the pain some women experience around menstruation. Prostaglandins, or other related substances, may also contribute to other negative somatic or mood changes.
3. A 'vulnerability' factor, which relates to a woman's general propensity for mood change. This may reflect both individual and constitutional characteristics as well as social or situational influences.

According to this model, women's experiences of menstrual cycle-related changes will reflect varying degrees of interaction between these three factors. If, for example, a woman has low 'vulnerability' and a minimal 'menstruation' factor, the 'timing' factor may be expressed relatively independently. This can be seen as the relatively normal cyclical process, affecting many but not all women and usually manifested as mild and manageable changes over the menstrual cycle.

If, on the other hand, this 'timing factor' operates in a woman with high 'vulnerability', for example a predisposition to depressive mood change, then we may expect to find this predisposition expressed at the stage of the hormonal cycle when the biochemical changes make her most vulnerable. Thus, on this basis the crucial difference between a woman who experiences severe premenstrual mood change and one who reports minimal or no cyclical mood change, lies not in the characteristics of their ovarian cycles, but in their general 'vulnerability'.

The 'menstruation' factor can operate in a comparable manner. In some women, changes involved in the menstrual process can result in adverse reactions which are confined to the menstrual phase of the cycle. If, however, these processes also interact with the effects of the 'timing factor', such women may experience more intense negative mood, both premenstrually and menstrually.

Let us consider each of these three factors more closely. The 'vulnerability' factor is perhaps most in need of clearer definition.

The Vulnerability Factor

Apart from 'neuroticism', which has already been mentioned, we also have to consider cognitive factors or cognitive 'style' which may render some women more susceptible to negative mood change. The application of cognitive therapy to women with PMS suggests that women with certain tendencies to depressive styles of thinking may be more prone to premenstrual mood change (Morse and Dennerstein, 1988).

Adverse events or problems in a woman's life may render her more vulnerable, eg. chronic marital problems or difficulties coping with children. There is only limited evidence of the role of stress as a moderating variable on menstrual cycle symptoms, although women attending PMS clinics often report that the severity of symptoms intensifies during periods of concurrent stress.

Biological markers of vulnerability may also be evident. It is noteworthy that the few recent studies which have found biological differences between women who experience perimenstrual depression and those who do not, have found these differences not restricted to the premenstrual phase but evident at all stages of the cycle which have been investigated. Thus, compared with controls, women with PMS have shown abnormalities in their neurendocrine responses to thyroid-releasing hormone (Roy-Byrne et al., 1987) and alterations in the pattern of melatonin secretion (Parry et al., 1990). In both of these cases the abnormalities were observed both in the early (follicular) and late (luteal) phases of the menstrual cycle.

We recently studied the neuroendocrine response to intravenous l-tryptophan, a dietary amino-acid (Bancroft et al., 1991). Normally, this biochemical challenge stimulates the pituitary to produce increased amounts of prolactin and growth hormone, as well as resulting in increased cortisol levels. In women suffering from a chronic depressive illness, these responses are blunted. Women with and without perimenstrual depression were tested on two occasions: premenstrually, when any depressive mood was likely to be at its peak, and postmenstrually, when in both groups mood would be relatively positive. Women with perimenstrual depression had blunted growth hormone and cortisol responses compared with the controls, but on *both* occasions ie. pre- and post-menstrually. On the other hand, the prolactin response was blunted only premenstrually but in *both groups of women*. This led us to postulate that some biochemical change in the brain occurs premenstrually in most women, accounting for the blunted prolactin response in both groups, but which in itself is insufficient to produce depressive mood change. The abnormal growth hormone and cortisol responses we attributed to a 'vulnerability' factor, although we do not yet know whether such abnormal responses would usually occur in these women (ie. a 'trait' phenomenon) or were only present during that particular cycle (ie. a 'state' phenomenon). However, the combination of this more persistent 'vulnerability' factor with the 'timing' factor might explain why they experienced their mood change during the premenstrual phase of that particular cycle.

The Timing Factor

What constitutes the 'timing' factor? As yet, our relevant evidence is extremely limited. In the above study, the prolactin response to L-tryptophan was altered premenstrually in women with and without cyclical mood changes. More research is required to pin down when such alteration in brain reactivity occurs and how it relates to the hormonal cycle. L-tryptophan is the precursor of 5-hydroxytryptamine (5-HT or serotonin), one of the key neurotransmitting catecholamines in the brain. The altered response to L-tryptophan suggests an alteration in 5-HT activity at that stage of the ovarian cycle. There is now considerable evidence implicating alteration of 5-HT activity in depressive illness. Interestingly, 5-HT is also implicated in the control of appetite. Increased carbohydrate intake results in an increased availability of tryptophan in the brain. A common premenstrual change is a craving for sweet foods. It has been postulated that premenstrual craving for sweet foods is an adaptive mechanism to compensate for the relative lack of 5-HT at that stage of the cycle.

In our study of women attending a gynaecology clinic with various complaints, described above, premenstrual food craving proved to be an interesting phenomenon. It was typically premenstrual in its timing. It was apparently unaffected by menstrual problems (ie. the 'menstruation' factor) and its association with neuroticism was low compared with its association with premenstrual emotional changes. Whilst it is commonly associated with premenstrual depression, premenstrual craving can occur on its own. Not only is it therefore of interest in its own right, it may also provide us with a marker of the cyclical changes in the brain, reflecting alteration in brain 5-HT activity, which is less susceptible than depressive mood change to other confounding factors. More research is required on this commonly-reported and potentially very interesting cyclical phenomenon.

It is generally assumed that any variation of brain function (eg. 5-HT activity) that underlies menstrual cycle-related mood change, is a function of varying levels of ovarian hormones. It is possible, for example, that the alteration of 5-HT activity is a consequence of falling levels of estradiol in the luteal phase of the cycle. We do not yet have the evidence to answer this question. But we should also consider another type of explanation. Is this cyclicity of brain function a form of entrained rhythm of brain activity, with the hormonal cycle simply determining the frequency of that rhythm? If so, this would explain why women using steroidal contraceptives often continue to experience a cyclical pattern of mood change which is indistinguishable from those accompanying normal ovarian cycles, in spite of their hormonal profile being very different (Walker and Bancroft, 1990). What is similar about a pill cycle and a 'normal' cycle is that it is imposing a roughly similar 'time-keeper', of about 28 days duration, on the brain. In a recent examination in which the ovarian cycle of women with PMS was disrupted by mifepristone, an antiprogestagen, so that their menstrual bleeding was induced earlier than otherwise would have happened, the cyclical symptoms occured at the time they should have done if bleeding had not been disrupted (Schmidt *et al.*, 1991). This suggested the persistence of an entrained rhythm of brain activity.

The Menstruation Factor

What do we know about the 'menstruation' factor? Mefenamic acid (Ponstan), which is a prostaglandin synthetase inhibitor, is used for the treatment of dysmenorrhoea and menorrhagia. It has also been shown to be beneficial for some premenstrual mood symptoms (Mira *et al.*, 1986). There is, therefore, some reason to believe that prostaglandins may be contributing to perimenstrual mood changes as well as physical complaints, although few studies have examined this possibility.

The effects of hysterectomy are also of interest. Removal of the uterus, leaving the ovaries intact, will result in the continuation of the ovarian hormonal cycle. To the extent that cyclical symptoms are dependent on this ovarian hormonal cycle, we should expect to find them continuing after hysterectomy, although less obviously because of the absence of the menstrual 'marker'. Several studies have shown this to be the case, although most have also reported that the severity of the symptoms are reduced after hysterectomy, suggesting that the uterus or the process of menstrual bleeding was contributing in some way to the severity of the cyclical mood changes. In a recent study, Metcalf and her colleagues (1991) found that persisting cyclical symptoms after hysterectomy reached their peak of severity significantly earlier than was the case in women with an intact uterus. They concluded that in some way the menstruation process either altered the timing of cyclical symptoms or made them more severe or prolonged. Once again, more research is required into the effects of menstruation on the premenstrual symptoms women experience.

Before concluding, let us reconsider how this 'three factor' model helps to explain the considerable variability of women's menstrual cycle experiences. The 'timing factor', as defined here, can be seen as a relatively normal phenomenon, though we must expect it to vary between women both in the extent of its impact on brain function and in its most obvious manifestations. For example, in some women, this variation in 5-HT activity may be more evident as appetite change, in others as mood change. Nevertheless we are postulating that this type of mechanism alone is unlikely to account for the severe problems that women attending PMS clinics typically report. The best term to describe this factor may need further debate and evidence; we are avoiding the term PMS because we believe it necessary to break from the medical and social constructs that have been associated with it.

When combined with some form of vulnerability, and we have acknowledged the varying forms this might take, then the 'timing factor' could result in the premenstrual timing of more severe types of mood change. In other words, the premenstrual phase may be the part of the cycle when the woman's vulnerability is going to be most readily manifested. As the 'vulnerability factor' gains in importance, the symptoms will be less restricted to the premenstrual phase of the cycle and progressively, negative mood will be evident at other phases of the woman's menstrual cycle, culminating in a typical depressive illness. Similarly, the 'menstruation factor' can be an additional influence, amplifying the mood changes both premenstrually and menstrually and blurring the more discrete premenstrual timing, attributable to the 'timing factor'.

This formulation not only sets a different agenda for clinical management of women presenting with perimenstrual complaints, with aspects of vulnerability and menstruation given more attention, but it also fundamentally alters the agenda for research in this area. Not only do we need to pursue the determinants of the 'timing factor' but the various forms of 'vulnerability' which are relevant need to be identified.

CONCLUSIONS

In this chapter, we have attempted to show the unsatisfactory nature of the concept of 'PMS' and have suggested an alternative model for managing and investigating cyclical mood change. This reappraisal has shifted emphasis away from 'abnormalities' of the menstrual cycle to viewing the hormonal cycle as linked to a fluctuating state of central nervous system reactivity which can interact with various types of vulnerability. Such vulnerabilities may be no different in men and women; what is different is that only women have this added effect of the menstrual cycle on brain function.

The nature of the relationship between the biological substrate of depressed mood (eg. alterations in 5-HT activity, or in the hypothalamic-pituitary-adrenal axis) and the psychosocial and cognitive determinants of depression is as yet obscure. Are they independent mechanisms, or are we observing a complex process of interaction with our environment through different windows – the neuroendocrine, the cognitive, the psychosocial? If so, are there constitutional differences in the biological stratum of this process which render women variable in their susceptibility to environmental challenges? And if so, are such constitutional differences between women, similar to those between men?

An important question is whether the recurrent provocation of negative mood associated with the menstrual cycle may increase the likelihood of a more sustained depressive illness. Such a question will be difficult to answer until longitudinal studies are carried out, and the various biological changes associated with perimenstrual changes and depressive illness are established as being of the 'state' or 'trait' variety.

In addition to grappling with the relationship between perimenstrual mood change and major depressive disorder, we need to integrate our findings and interpretations of such effects of the menstrual cycle with our understanding of the effects on mood and well-being of other aspects of women's reproductive status ie. their reactions to pregnancy and the puerperium, to steroidal contraceptives and to the hormonal changes of the perimenopause. In all respects we must strive to understand how the biological interacts with the cognitive and the psychosocial.

Finally, more attention should be paid to the positive menstrual cycle-related changes which some women experience. Sanders *et al.* (1983) found a postmenstrual 'elevation' in mood in women with premenstrual depression which was not evident in women without such premenstrual worsening of mood. As we have discussed, positive cyclical changes have received little research attention and yet this postmenstrual elevated mood may be as important a phenomenon to study as the premenstrual mood decline if we are to gain a better understanding of cyclical mood change.

FURTHER READING

Asso, D. (1983). *The real menstrual cycle*. Chichester: Wiley.

Bancroft, J. and Backstrom, T. (1985). Premenstrual syndrome. *Clinical Endocrinology*, 22, 313–336.

Dan, A.J. and Lewis, L.L. (Eds.) (1992). *Menstrual health in women's lives*. Chicago: University of Illinois Press.

Ginsburg, B.E. and Carter, B.F. (Eds.) (1987) *Premenstrual syndrome. Ethical and legal implications in a biomedical perspective*. New York: Plenum.

3

REPRODUCTIVE ISSUES: DECISIONS AND DISTRESS

MARIE JOHNSTON

Department of Psychology, University of St. Andrews, St. Andrews KY16 9AJ, Scotland, UK

Reproductive issues offer women considerable satisfaction as well as the challenge of choosing and deciding the best personal course, and the worry and uncertainties of the outcomes. This chapter focuses on two psychological issues: the decision processes involved and the emotional distress. These two are chosen, first because they permeate most reproductive processes, second because they affect most women in some way and third because there is a large literature on these topics over a wide range of reproductive concerns.

A limited set of reproductive issues have been selected: pregnancy, screening during pregnancy, abortion, infertility, labor and childbirth. Again, the selection has been of common issues affecting many women and with substantial research literatures. Therefore, issues which affect a small proportion of women such as fetal loss, having a handicapped child and postnatal depression are not discussed.

Much of the evidence discussed comes from studies of women in medical settings. Inevitably this gives a bias to the information that is available – after all, most reproductive experiences do not occur in a medical setting. However, the development of medical techniques for overcoming infertility and reducing the hazards of pregnancy, abortion, infertility, labor and childbirth. Again, the selection has been of and other health care professionals in matters which families dealt with in previous generations.

Men's roles have been largely ignored because women are the focus of this book, but also because more is known about women's responses and experiences. Relationship issues are only minimally discussed because an adequate discussion would require reproductive issues to be addressed in a much wider context.

DECISION PROCESSES

Many reproductive issues offer women the opportunity to make a decision and choose between outcomes. Psychological models used to explain other behaviors, including health behaviors, can be applied to reproductive behaviors and models such as Subjective Expected Utility, the Theory of Reasoned Action, the Theory of Planned Behavior or the Health Belief Model incorporate rational decision making in the explanatory process. These rational decisions are postulated to depend on beliefs about the behaviors involved, about threats associated with action or inaction, about the likely outcomes of behavior, about the opinions of other people and so on. In examining reproductive decisions, evidence is sought for such beliefs which might form the basis of the decision, although the existence of such beliefs does not necessarily imply that they informed the decision as they may simply be post hoc rationalizations.

Other decision models do not require such a simple rational process. Conflict Theory puts more emphasis on the choice between opposing alternatives and the emotion generated is seen to influence the outcome. Weinstein's (1988) Precaution Adoption Process envisages stages of decision making, not all of which involve rational processes. This model might be applied to contraceptive behaviors or to steps the woman may take to avoid being childless. The early stages in the process, recognizing a risk exists, becoming aware of one's personal risk and deciding to take action are most likely to be influenced by the rational processes described in the Theory of Reasoned Action. Whereas the final stage, taking precautionary action, does not appear to be influenced by conscious rational processes according to evidence available to date (Weinstein, 1988). These models may help to explain why women who do not wish to become pregnant, do, and why women who intend to have infertility treatment delay in seeking help.

Where a woman engages in a behavior such as becoming pregnant or having a screening test, it does not necessarily follow that she has made a *reproductive* decision. She may have made a social decision, eg. to do what every other woman does, or a self-protective decision, eg. to avoid pain. If so, then there is less likely to be evidence of supportive reproductive beliefs, although there may be other supportive beliefs.

When a woman makes these decisions, she is frequently making them in some social situation, especially with her sexual partner, her family or her medical advisers. To understand her decisions fully, one would need to examine the behavior of these other people too, but they are largely ignored in the current chapter, as the focus here is on the woman herself.

Pregnancy

The reasons women give for wanting to have a baby include liking children, seeking immortality, raising their self-esteem and being like other women. However, women do not necessarily make decisions about becoming pregnant and having a baby. Instead, reproductive outcomes may be determined by decisions in other domains such as choice of dating partner, whether to avoid risk of HIV infection, how much alcohol to drink etc.

A current major area of study of reproductive decision making is that of teenage pregnancies, particularly in the US. The frequency of these pregnancies, especially in deprived social groups, and the resulting abortions and/or associated social problems, has led to a significant investment of research funds. Research in the UK found that pregnant 16–19 year olds had good knowledge of contraception (Phoenix, 1989). The 79 women had the following orientations to pregnancy:

wanted to conceive	22%
did not mind	25%
had not thought about it	18%
important not to conceive	35%

Of the 28 women who had considered it important not to become pregnant, 17 had used no contraception. Amongst the reasons given for not using contraception were: difficulties in obtaining and storing contraception, attitudes to methods available including concerns about effects on their health of the pill and lack of trust in the sheath, belief that they would not become pregnant, beliefs that men were less concerned about using contraceptives, and not taking control of contraception early in their sexual careers or in new sexual relationships.

One might expect the decision process to be clearer for women who have problems in conception and pregnancy. Women who had a high risk in pregnancy, either to their own health due to congenital cardiac defects or to the fetus due to a history of miscarriages, have been found to be more likely to have planned their pregnancies than those with normal risk. However, having a child was no more important to them as a life goal than for women having an unthreatened pregnancy (Bielawska-Batorowicz, 1990).

Having become pregnant, the woman may have to make various decisions about changing her lifestyle for the sake of the fetus's health. In particular, she may have to make decisions about giving up smoking, diet, drug ingestion and alcohol intake as they are associated with the birth of babies who are at risk due to low birthweight. The women discussed above who had high risk pregnancies, were more likely to change their lifestyle than women at normal risk. Women are more likely to change their habits if they believe that they have control over the fetus's health. Using the Fetal Health Locus of Control Scale (FHLC), a questionnaire developed to measure expectancies for locus of control beliefs, women who gave up smoking had higher scores on internal FHLC than non-quitters and beliefs in chance locus of control were associated with continuing to smoke (Labs and Wurtele, 1986). Those with internal FHLC were also more likely to reduce their caffeine intake.

Attendance at antenatal classes is also predictive of good pregnancy outcomes. Women's scores on the internal FHLC was the only significant predictor of intention to attend prepared childbirth classes in a discriminant function analysis (Labs and Wurtele, 1986). Other studies of women having their first baby have shown that intention to attend antenatal classes is related to their attitudes to antenatal classes, in particular to the extent to which they believe that the costs of attending outweigh the benefits (Michie *et al.*, 1990). Intention to attend was the best predictor of actual attendance.

The research in this area has shown a clearer focus in examining the decisions of women once they are pregnant. The importance of the woman's behavior in determining the outcome for the fetus, as well as the ease of studying women in obstetric departments, has resulted in some advance in theoretical and empirical research in this area. By contrast, only a small amount is known about the decision processes that result in pregnancy, perhaps because this has only relatively recently been seen as a decision. Other important decisions in pregnancy are considered under other headings.

Abortion

Women who are unhappy about being pregnant may make a decision to continue with the pregnancy or to abort the baby. Many women who continue with a pregnancy, despite initially being unhappy about it have been found to change their attitudes during pregnancy and show more favorable attitudes by the final three months (Wolkind and Zajicek, 1981). However, this does not indicate that those who have an abortion would also go on to change how they feel.

A large proportion of pregnancies are aborted. A recent review of abortion in the US found that the majority of women having abortions are under 25 and unmarried (Adler *et al.*, 1990). Most women having an abortion report that they did not find the decision difficult. For women having an abortion within the first three months of pregnancy, only 12 percent were found to have difficulty in making the decision, although this number rises to 51 percent in those having a late abortion, the delay presumably being the result of the indecision. Women are more likely to be satisfied with their decision if they perceive that they have support for their decision from those around them and if they have a favorable attitude toward abortion in general terms. The decision process has implications, not only at the time of the abortion when it may lead to indecision and delay, but later, after the abortion, the level of psychological distress is related to difficulties in making the decision (Adler *et al.*, 1990).

Some abortions are undertaken for medical reasons including both the health of the woman and a diagnosed defect in the child. For most women, this decision is more likely to be a decision to accept medical advice than to weigh the pros and cons of continuing with the pregnancy. The decision about abortion is influenced by many different individual beliefs, including religious beliefs and beliefs about the acceptability of abortion. As abortion has become a more popular choice, it will be important to evaluate the extent to which social and cultural beliefs about the acceptability of abortion and about the value of an imperfect fetus are affected by the frequency of the practice. Comparison of countries where abortion rates differ might inform this question. In the small number of cases where a woman decides to continue with a pregnancy where the fetus carries a diagnosed defect such as Down's syndrome, this can create tensions for the clinical obstetric team and for the woman at the time of delivery.

Where the medical advice is more ambivalent as when the fetus carries a risk but not a certainly of an impairment, the woman and her partner may be involved in highly complex decision making where they are presented with probability values for each possible outcome. Specialists in genetic medicine frequently recognize the problems involved and attempt to overcome them by presenting the couple with as complete information as possible. However, there is ample evidence that people make poor use of such information (eg. Shiloh and Saxe, 1989) and that doctors make significant errors in handling probability data. Thus, the likelihood of a 'rational', information-based decision is low and the nature of these decisions remains to be researched.

Infertility

Perhaps the clearest reproductive decision is demonstrated by women who seek medical assistance to become pregnant. It is difficult to assess what proportion of couples, who do not conceived spontaneously, consult with infertility problems. Not all childless couples are infertile, but even amongst those who are, not all seek medical help. The research evidence is biassed towards studies of those who present at infertility clinics and little is known of the decisions of those who do not seek help.

Women are much more likely to present with problems of infertility than are their partners. A curious by-product of this behavioral bias is that medical science is considerably better informed about the human female reproductive system than about the male as more women have been available for study. As a result, more treatment options have been developed which involve the woman, thereby reinforcing the value of the woman consulting.

Studies of women seeking infertility treatment (see Adler *et al.*, 1991), suggest that this involves a positive decision to achieve reproduction, but a few women report being involved in the investigation and treatment process almost as part of a natural progression or a normal social process, rather than as the result of a decision about the importance of having a child. The process of medical care rarely involves consideration of the reproductive decision process, concentrating instead on infertility as a biological impairment. As one woman, who had completed years of infertility investigations, responded to a research question about reasons for wanting a baby, "I thought no one would ever ask me that".

A major question about deciding to engage in infertility treatment concerns the quality of the information available to the woman and her partner, especially information about the likely success of the procedures. Simple subjective expected utility models predict that decisions are made on the basis of the value of the expected outcome and the likelihood of that outcome. For decisions to engage in infertility treatment, one needs to consider not only the value the woman places on having a baby, but also her perception of the likelihood of success of the treatment procedure. Clearly, if the value of a baby is extremely high, the woman may engage in the procedure even with a low expectation of success.

However, there may be some who become involved in treatment because they are overoptimistic about their likely success. There is now a large body of evidence that women deciding to have in vitro fertilisation (IVF) overestimate the chances of success. Given a live birth rate of generally less than 15 percent for each attempt, estimates of success given by individual patients range from less than 10 per cent to over 80 percent in studies in New Zealand, UK and US (Adler *et al.*, 1991). Figure 3.1 illustrates the range of responses in one study (Johnston *et al.*, 1987).

The staff of clinics may inadvertently contribute to this overestimation. At the simplest level, their active engagement in the treatment procedures may imply that they are very successful, and even though the staff attempt to explain the limited success, action may speak louder than words. Also, the much publicised pictures of clinicians with IVF babies presents an image of success. This combined with the media bias of presenting successful IVF rather than the less newsworthy as well as less easily illustrated failure, results in women receiving a biassed version of the success rates. We have suggested that this bias combined with the known tendency to estimate the probability of events according to the number we can bring to mind (the availability heuristic) may account for the overestimation involved (Johnston, *et al.*, 1987).

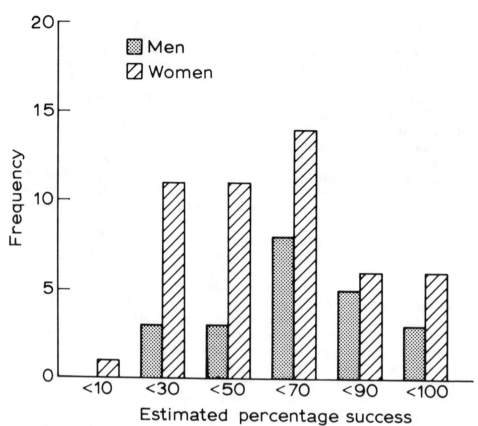

FIGURE 3.1   *Estimates of likely success of IVF. Johnston et al., 1987.*

An alternative explanation is that the overestimation of success is part of a coping process which makes the stress of undergoing IVF procedures more tolerable. If so, then the overestimation should be confined to those having IVF. However, this is not the case; in a study of a nonclinical sample, 89 percent of students overestimated the likely success of IVF (Adib, 1988). In an analysis of factors contributing to optimism about IVF in women on the waiting list for IVF after completing initial assessment procedures, women's knowledge about IVF was the only significant predictive variable in a multiple regression analysis and other independent variables (anxiety, self-esteem, marital harmony and time on the waiting list) did not add to the prediction (Johnston *et al.*, 1990). It would therefore appear that information and biases may contribute to a greater expectation of success than is valid, at the time of making the decision to have IVF.

One still needs to ask whether this optimism about success influences the decision to engage in IVF procedures. Information about the estimates of success of IVF by eligible women who refuse to participate would be useful but is not available. However, some evidence is available about participation or non-participation in a second treatment cycle, following an initial failure. Lack of success of the procedure was given as the second most important reason for not pursuing a second attempt, costs being the most important. It is therefore highly possible that overestimation of success encourages women to undergo IVF procedures.

Screening in Pregnancy

Some of the tests in pregnancy which screen for fetal abnormalities are done routinely ie. they are offered to all women, eg. ultrasound scanning, AFP screening for neural tube defects and Down's syndrome. Women who do not have the AFP test fall into two groups, those who decline the test and those who simply omit to have the test (Marteau *et al.*, 1992). Those who omitted to have the test had less knowledge about the test than those who had it, while those who declined the test had more negative attitudes toward termination of an affected fetus, more negative attitudes toward doctors and medicine, perceived the threat of an abnormal child to be less and had less knowledge of the screening test. These results suggest that the first group of women may not be engaged in a decision process and may even fail to be offered the test in the clinic, whereas those who decline appear to have made an active decision to opt out of the routine care on the basis of a consistent value system.

Other tests are offered only if the pregnancy is at increased risk, for example due to increased maternal age, due to abnormal levels on the AFP test or due to problems apparent in earlier pregnancies. The most investigated of these tests is amniocentesis screening for chromosomal abnormalities, especially in women over 35 years of age. In centers where amniocentesis is available, uptake rates in eligible women vary greatly from one area to another. These variations may reflect the local processes involved in the test becoming safer, more acceptable and more routine, as it has also been observed that uptake rates at one clinic increase with time. Compared with women who have the test, women who do not tend to view the risks of having an abnormal fetus as greater and would be less likely to consider a termination if the fetus were affected. The woman's perception of her risk of carrying an affected child is a better predictor of uptake of amniocentesis than is her actual risk, as indicated by her age (Marteau *et al.*, 1991).

The emphasis of current research in this area has shifted from the individual beliefs of the women to the communication process between the woman and the health care team. Unlike decisions about pregnancy and abortion, the relevant information about screening tests is not necessarily gathered in the social network outside the clinic, especially as they depend on very recent developments in medical research. Insofar as decisions depend on information gained in the clinic, it will be necessary to obtain further details about the interactions between the woman and those giving her information and advice.

Labor

When asked 6 weeks after the birth 'in general, did you feel in control of what staff were doing to you during labor?', the percentage of replies of 656 women were:

(Green, 1990a)

yes, always	27
yes, most of the time	53
only some of the time	14
no, hardly at all	7

The main decisions that woman may have control over and which have been researched are those concerning use of analgesia during labor. It has been suggested that two main motivations determine this decision: avoidance of pain, and avoidance of anaesthesia. When asked their preferences, women early in labor chose to avoid anaesthesia whereas at a later stage, during active labor, they preferred to avoid pain (Christensen-Szalanski, 1984). One month later, their preference shifted toward avoiding anaesthesia. While this was a small study of 18 women enrolled in a class that stressed childbirth without the use of anaesthesia, the results point to the importance of investigating the decision processes at the appropriate time. They also indicate sources of dissatisfaction with the chosen decision as women have a different preference after the event compared with during late labor.

It is only recently that research on patient choice of medical treatment has been conducted and one can expect more research in this area. As in other areas of medical care, it is difficult to estimate how much control the woman has over decisions that are taken unless this is explicitly defined for a research study.

DISTRESS

There is a bias in all psychological studies towards distress rather than more positive emotions. Thus, psychologists have evolved satisfactory measures of anxiety, depression, anger, negative affect etc. but have given relatively little attention to happiness, joy, serenity and other positive emotions. Where positive emotion measures are developed, they have often been criticized for measuring little other than the absence of negative emotions, but enough evidence exists to suggest that there may be some independence and that it would be unwise to equate lack of negative emotion with joy.

This bias is well founded if one observes the functions of psychology. Given the major role in understanding and reducing distress, it has been essential to develop measures and theoretical models. If psychologists were commissioned to promote joy and fulfillment, these processes might be more satisfactorily researched. The bias is also consistent with the practice of medicine concerning reproductive issues. Doctors spend a disproportionate amount of time with, and are most likely to engage the help of psychologists to work with women who are having difficulties and are thus more likely to be distressed.

As noted above, women are more likely to present with reproductive problems than are men and many medical procedures concerning obstetrics and fertility can be undertaken with only the woman present. As a result, most evidence is available about women's distress.

Important theoretical perspectives that need to be considered are models of stress and of individual differences. Many reproductive events can be seen as stressors: some are threats, eg. of miscarriage or of having an abnormal baby, while others are losses, eg. of a wanted baby or of the freedom of childlessness, and the birth of a baby may be seen as a challenge. It is noteworthy that models of life stress and transitions and measures of life events typically give considerable prominence to such issues.

The interaction between psychological and physiological stress processes is also important in understanding the relationship between the woman's emotions and the biological changes involved. There are many areas where it is virtually impossible to disentangle the causal pathways. For example, at what point does the distress associated with being infertile result in hormonal changes which might interfere with normal fertilization (Edelman and Golombok, 1989), or is there a level of psychological disturbances which may be the primary cause of infertility? Similarly, does anxiety about going into premature labor result in neuroendocrine processes which induce premature labor, and surely the threat of premature labor is sufficient to increase anxiety levels. It is important to investigate both directions of causality.

Individual difference models can also make an important contribution to understanding distress concerning reproductive issues. Transient states of high anxiety in response to events may be due to the objective stressfulness of the events; or they may be explained to some extent by individual differences in trait anxiety, the disposition to develop high levels of state anxiety in response to threatening events, whether they are relevant to reproduction or not. Women who describe their experiences as being highly worrying or distressing may have experienced more threatening or bad outcomes; alternatively, they may be displaying high individual levels of 'negative affectivity', the tendency to interpret events in a negative light, and such women would see the negative side of many experiences.

In addition to trait anxiety and negative affectivity, women may differ in their predominant coping styles, in their levels of perceived control over events and in their perceived social support. A contrast has been made between avoidant and attentional coping styles. Someone with an avoidant coping style directs their attention away from threat, whereas the person with an attentional style directs their attention to threat. Evidence to date (Suls and Fletcher, 1985) suggests that an avoidant style is adaptive in dealing with short-term stressors such as labor or IVF surgery, whereas an attentional style is more successful for enduring stresses such as infertility. Perceived control has been examined in a number of ways, but important contrasts have been made between perceiving events to be influenced by one's own behavior (internal control), by the behavior of powerful others and by chance events outside anyone's control. While internal control has frequently been associated with less distress, this may not be the case when things go wrong and in a medical setting where considerable control is exercised by health professionals, belief in control by powerful others may be useful. Finally, women may differ in the degree of social support which they perceive to be available and this has been found to be extremely important both in predicting emotional well-being in general and when people are subject to life stresses.

Pregnancy

In popular culture, becoming pregnant and having a child is seen as a source of joy and fulfillment for women. When one turns to psychological studies of the process, one finds a much greater focus on anxiety and worries. Early in pregnancy, one study found that 74 percent of the women described themselves as happy about it, but 46 percent were anxious and had worries about the possibility of a miscarriage, something being wrong with baby, money, being in hospital, internal examinations etc. (Green, 1990b). Anxiety is found to be commoner later in pregnancy and it has been suggested that this may be due to having more realistic expectations of labor and the birth. While many of those who were upset about being pregnant in the early stages were more positive by 7 months, some who were initially happy to be pregnant became more negative (Wolkind and Zajicek, 1981). Women who already have a child tend to be more anxious than those having a first baby, confirming the suggestion above that additional information about late pregnancy and birth tends to raise rather than lower anxiety.

Women who have had previous reproductive problems, such as a miscarriage, are also more anxious. Nevertheless, a study of overall mood during pregnancy found that 72 percent reported that they were 'reasonably cheerful most of the time' (Green, 1990b).

High levels of anxiety during pregnancy are important both for the welfare of the fetus and for the mother's postnatal mental health, in addition to the immediate distress experienced by the women. Anxiety in pregnancy is related to poor growth in the fetus, complications around the time of birth and problems in the subsequent relationship between the mother and her baby (Reading, 1983; Istvan, 1986). There are several possible explanations. First, the mother's anxiety may affect the fetus directly through neuroendocrine processes, eg. increased levels of catecholamines may cause placental insufficiency resulting in both premature delivery and low birthweight. Second, high anxiety may encourage the mother to take alcohol, anxiety-reducing drugs or to smoke more and this may indirectly affect the fetus's health. Third, anxiety during labor may adversely affect progress, both by limiting her ability to participate and as a result of neuroendocrine processes.

Women who are highly anxious late in pregnancy are more likely to show clinical levels of postnatal depression and it has been suggested that programs designed to reduce the incidence of postnatal depression should target women who are particularly distressed in the last three months of pregnancy. Such evidence as exists indicates that unmarried mothers are no more likely than married or cohabiting women to become seriously distressed in pregnancy, but there is a tendency for teenage mothers to be more vulnerable than older mothers (see Niven, 1992).

Pregnancy can be considered as a life stressor which requires a considerable degree of adaptation. In addition, it changes the pattern of the woman's relationships, especially with her partner and it has been suggested that the balance changes from one where the woman gives more social support to one where she needs more than her partner. Social support is a particularly important resource to the pregnant woman, especially if she is experiencing a high level of life events and psychological distress; such women have been found to be more likely to have complications in pregnancy if they lack social support. In one study, the level of professional support was increased for women at risk of having a low birthweight baby. Compared with a control group, those having this increased support had heavier babies and also had increased support from friends and family (see Niven, 1992).

Screening in Pregnancy

In addition to the stresses inherent in pregnancy, women now have the additional stress of tests which screen for abnormalities in the fetus. These tests not only carry the possibility of producing distressing results, they may threaten the viability of the fetus and on occasion may incur some risk to the mother herself. They can also be reassuring. However, where women have been found to show reduced anxiety following a test, it is frequently unclear whether the woman has been reassured or if the results have simply dispelled the anxiety raised by having the test. Women have been found to show false reassurance, generalizing from the results of a test for a single condition to the belief that the baby was healthy in all ways. For routine screening for neural tube defects by a blood test, some women have been found to be unaware that they had had the test and were therefore unlikely to have been reassured.

A very small proportion of women will have an impairment in the fetus diagnosed and will therefore have received a 'positive' result. For most women, the results of screening tests will be negative and even for most of those receiving a positive result, subsequent testing will show that result to be false. Women receiving a false positive result show high levels of anxiety. Using standard measures of anxiety, women having a positive screening blood test result, but later found to have a negative result, had anxiety levels approaching those of psychiatric patients with generalized anxiety disorder (Robinson *et al.*, 1984). Anxiety normally reduces when they receive the negative second result, but some of these women continue to have high levels of anxiety and the method of communicating the result can affect the degree of anxiety-reduction. The anxiety raised by a false positive result does not necessarily dissipate quickly and in some studies women have continued to experience heightened anxiety late in pregnancy and to report concern about the baby's health even some weeks after birth.

Abortion

There has been considerable concern that the abortion of an unwanted pregnancy may be stressful in itself and might therefore result in emotional disturbance in the woman. Responses after an abortion are a composite of the experience of the unwanted pregnancy, the decision to have an abortion and the physical ordeal. A recent review concludes that the evidence to date indicates that an early legal abortion of an unwanted pregnancy "does not pose a psychological hazard for most women." (Adler *et al.*, 1990). Two weeks afterwards, 76 percent of women have been found to report relief, with only 17 percent reporting feeling guilt, and positive emotions typically outweigh negative emotions. A comparison of pregnant adolescents who had an abortion with those who gave birth to the baby found that two years later the abortion group had lower trait anxiety and a higher sense of internal control than the birth group, suggesting that the abortion had not been as damaging as having the baby would have been.

Women who do show negative psychological responses have been found to be more likely to have intended to become pregnant and to have found the decision to have an abortion difficult. Where the indecision has resulted in a later abortion, it is likely that the physical trauma is greater than in an early abortion, so that physical stressors add to the psychological stress. Research on support available suggests that women with more social support for the abortion from parents and partner show more positive responses. Women who expected to cope well showed less evidence of depression than those with negative expectations, while women using an avoidant coping strategy prior to the abortion showed more anxiety and depression afterwards than those using an attentional strategy. In sum, the existing research evidence suggests that those who continue to be distressed after the abortion are those who have not resolved ambivalent feelings prior to the abortion; this conclusion is supported by the finding that women randomly allocated to receive pre-abortion counselling based on coping and attributional theories were less depressed after the abortion than those receiving standard counselling.

Infertility

Emotional problems associated with infertility have only been studied in those women presenting to a doctor and then only after the infertility has been of considerable duration. Thus it is difficult to interpret results obtained as either the cause or consequence of the infertility. Results are not consistent in reporting high levels of emotional and marital disturbance in women having infertility investigations and treatment (Connolly *et al.*, 1987). This result is surprising, given that the continuing high levels of effort and time invested, the discomforts of the procedures, and the uncertainty of the outcomes might have been expected to contribute to high levels of distress in themselves. An attempt to separate out these different sources of stress compared women who had had a baby as a result of infertility treatment with spontaneously fertile women. The former were consistently less satisfied with health and life, had less life happiness and were more depressed (Bromham *et al.*, 1989). One might interpret these results as showing either the cumulative effects of the stresses involved or the distress and dissatisfaction with life of those entering infertility treatment. However, this was a cross-sectional study on a small sample with only about a 33 percent response rate.

As the range of possible investigations and treatments increases with developments in medical technology, more women will successfully overcome infertility problems. On the other hand, more women will go through longer periods of unsuccessful medical attention. Studies of patients having IVF treatments show that they are anxious at the time of having the procedures, as might be expected of those having a surgical procedure or any procedure with an uncertain outcome (Johnston *et al.*, 1987). The most commonly cited negative aspects of the experience of IVF treatment has been found to be the interactions with health-care professionals, but these interactions were also the source of the most positive outcomes.

Follow-up studies of IVF patients have resulted in low response rates from those who were unsuccessful (Adler *et al.*, 1991). As a result, it is almost impossible to interpret the findings. Some studies find emotional distress levels within the normal range, while others find evidence of higher rates of disturbance and yet others find low rates. However, those responding in any particular study may be biassed toward those who have made the better psychological adjustment or toward those who are still most distressed and wishing for continued contact with the clinic.

Because of the difficulties inherent in research in this area, some authors have suggested that future research should not be oriented toward the assessment of distress and disturbance but to understanding the coping styles and strategies which are most effective in dealing with the stresses involved.

Labor

Labor is associated with high levels of pain and associated anxiety, and anticipation of the pain is a source of intense anxiety for many pregnant women. Using a standardized pain measure, pain during labor has been found to exceed that associated with back pain, cancer, phantom limbs, toothache and arthritis, especially in the later stages of labor (see figure 3.2; Niven and Gijsbers, 1984). While reports of pain severity vary between studies, a study in Scotland found that only 8 percent of women reported very little pain whereas 16 percent rated the pain "as bad as I could possibly imagine" (Niven, 1986).

Labor pain has been found to be higher in women having a first baby, in younger women and in those of low social class, but these associations are not reliably found. Women experiencing more pain early on in labor are more likely to have a Caesarian

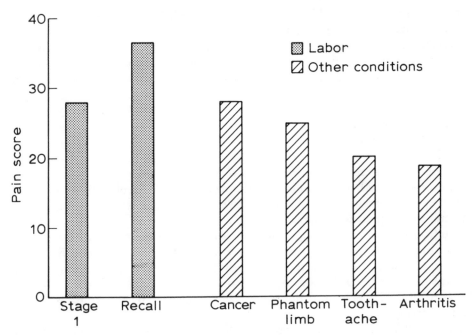

FIGURE 3.2 Pain in labor compared with other clinical pain. Niven and Gijsbers, 1984.

section, to have Pethidine as analgesia and to have babies who have problems with breathing.

Pregnant women show considerable concern about coping with labor. Those who attend antenatal classes have been shown to be more confident about it following the class (Hiller and Slade, 1989). They were also more knowledgeable, but the level of knowledge varied with the class the women had attended. The more classes the woman attended the less her overall anxiety, but anxiety and knowledge were not related.

When questioned 6 weeks after the birth about their feelings during labor, in a cohort of 660 women 41 percent reported being 'frightened', 18 percent 'out of control' and 18 percent 'helpless'. Only 23 percent reported feeling 'confident' and 'in control' (Green, 1990b). While one might question such retrospective data, other evidence indicates that women recall labor experiences clearly. Women who had given birth 3 to 4 years previously reported similar qualitative and quantitative pain experiences to those actually reported at the time of delivery (Niven, 1988).

There is some evidence that the pain experienced can be influenced by the coping strategies the woman uses. Pain reported during labor was less in women who reported using a variety of coping strategies; these included relaxation, breathing techniques, distraction and re-interpretation of the pain in a more positive way and were used by 33, 75, 67 and 22 percent of the 51 women (Niven, 1986). The more strategies the woman used, the lower the levels of pain reported.

A number of studies show that preparation for childbirth, especially training in relaxation and breathing exercises, results in less pain and discomfort, and reduced use of analgesia, although there are studies which show no positive benefits (see Adler *et al.*, 1990). These results are similar to those obtained in preparing patients for surgical or painful medical procedures.

Social support during labor may also be beneficial. Women in premature labor randomly allocated to receive additional help from a supporter trained to give support, information and relaxation training were found to have shorter labor, use less analgesic medication and have improved neonatal well-being compared with the control group (Cogan and Spinnato, 1988). Factors affecting labor pain are discussed further in Chapter 4.

CONCLUSIONS

Decisions and distress about reproductive issues have been widely researched. However, some methodological problems are common to much of this research. First, it is frequently impossible to obtain a sample which is unbiassed and results can be difficult to interpret. Second, many studies use retrospective research designs due to the difficulty of questioning women at the time of key decisions or of high distress, and results may be colored by subsequent experiences or the woman's state at the time of reporting. Third, much of the research depends on self-report measures which can be misleading; the data may be biassed due to poor recall, due to individual styles such as negative affectivity or due to the report being influenced by the woman's current coping strategy.

Nevertheless, there are some consistent patterns emerging with a variety of samples, research designs and methods, which provide empirical evidence about these decisions and distress. This is important in advising women, in guiding medical practice and in planning psychological interventions which may facilitate decision making and reduce unnecessary distress. For example, the evidence to date suggests that there is little long-term adverse effect of abortion in those women who make the decision easily. This is useful information at the time of such decisions and suggests that interventions might be designed, based on decision analysis models or involving social support functions, to assist the decisions of those finding the decision difficult.

Current scientific advances, particularly in analyzing the human genome, are likely to result in the development of more medical technologies, requiring more decisions and probably resulting in more distress for the women involved. The last ten years have seen the development of many new tests for the detection of disorders of the fetus and these have been implemented in obstetric care allowing the choice of whether to terminate or continue the pregnancy. Tests are being developed which will be applied prior to pregnancy to indicate whether an individual or a couple carry an increased risk of having a child with certain genetic defects such as Huntington's Chorea or Cystic Fibrosis. Similarly, increased understanding of the processes of fertilization and pregnancy has resulted in many new treatments for infertility.

These new reproductive technologies offer new opportunities to overcome problems. But they also impose new burdens: decisions concerning the use of the procedure, discomfort or even risk in undergoing the process and uncertainties about the likely success of the techniques.

In addition to providing the opportunity for health psychology to offer useful applied and applicable information, research on reproductive decisions and distress allows the possibility of developing psychological theory. Theories of stress and coping, typically examine both emotion-focussed and problem-focussed coping and could clearly encompass investigations of both decisions and distress. Theories of health related behaviors allows reproductive behaviors to be seen in the context of other health behaviors. There are signs that this research field is gradually being influenced by theoretical models developed in other areas. Perhaps this will become more of a reciprocal relationship in the future, with research on reproductive issues contributing more to basic psychological theory.

FURTHER READING

Adler, N.E., David, H.P., Major, B.N., Roth, S.H., Russo, N.F. and Wyatt, G.E. (1990). Psychological responses after abortion. *Science*, **248**, 41–44.

Adler, N.E., Keyes, S. and Robertson, P. (1991). Psychological issues in new reproductive technologies: pregnancy-inducing technology and diagnostic screening. In J. Rodin and A. Collins (Eds.) *Women and new reproductive technologies: Medical, psychosocial, legal and ethical dilemmas*. Hillsdale, NJ: Lawrence Erlbaum.

Marteau, T.M., Johnston, M., Kidd, J., Michie, S., Cook, R., Slack, J. and Shaw, R.W. (1992). Psychological models in predicting uptake of prenatal screening. *Psychology and Health*, **6**, 13–22.

Niven, C. (1992). *Psychological care for families: before, during and after birth*. Oxford: Butterworth Heinemann.

4

WOMEN AND THE EXPERIENCE OF PAIN

KAREL GIJSBERS

Department of Psychology, University of Stirling, Stirling FK0 4LA, Scotland, UK

CATHERINE A. NIVEN

Department of Psychology, Glasgow Polytechnic, Cowcaddens Road, Glasgow G4 0BA, Scotland, UK

It is difficult to discuss pain as experienced by women without contrasting their perception of pain with that of men. One of the more reproducible phenomenon in studies of experimental pain is a sex difference in pain thresholds and tolerance. Differences also occur in studies of incidence of clinical pain. Women seem to be more sensitive to experimentally induced pain as well as being more likely than men to report incidences of clinical pain. Are women then, more prone to pain? And if they are, why should this be? Is it the consequence of differences in the physiological mechanisms mediating pain, secondary consequences of differences in illness rate, or is it related in some way to differences in gender role expectations? The pain experience of women is almost certainly influenced by their reproductive capacities. Women from puberty may experience pain associated with menstruation, and most women experience quite high levels of pain during childbirth. After giving birth, women sometimes have to deal with pain associated with episiotomy or breast feeding. These experiences of pain, unique to women, could influence their perception of other pains not specifically related to reproduction. Women also tend to report pains whose organic origins are obscure (eg. Repetition Strain Injury or Irritable Bowel Syndrome, see later discussion) which can involve them in complex interactions with the medical profession who may not always believe that they are suffering (Reid *et al.*, 1991). Consequently, the pain of women may be exacerbated by the need to persuade doctors, nurses, etc. that their pain reports are credible. Overall, a range of factors exist which could predispose women to be characterized as the 'suffering' sex.

We intend in this chapter to focus on the evidence for differences between the sexes in their pain perception and experience, and to discuss the particular significance that pain related to reproduction may have for women. Unfortunately the results of clinical and experimental studies of pain are often complex and sometimes contradictory. Since our discussion should be physiologically plausible, we provide in the initial section of our discussion, an outline of the mechanisms in the peripheral nervous system and spinal cord that are thought to mediate pain.

PAIN MECHANISMS

The brain can be subdivided into the two cerebral hemispheres and its core, the brainstem which extends outside the skull as the spinal cord. The cerebral hemispheres, the brainstem and spinal cord make up the central nervous system whose functioning depends on the electrical activity of neuron cells which are distinguished by being able systematically to modify each other's electrical activity. Neurons are composed of an axon that transmits information in the form of electrical activity from one cell to another, a cell body or soma that is sensitive to activation by the axons of other neurons, and dendrites; processes which in effect extend the receptive surface of the cell body to axonal input. The central nervous system is subdivided into distinctive nuclei or clusters of neuronal cell bodies and fibre tracts consisting of axons that carry information between the neuronal clusters. The peripheral nervous system also consists of neurons that project into and from the spinal cord. These neurons are responsible for the control of glands, viscera and skeletal muscles, and for transmitting information to the spinal cord from a variety of sensory 'receptors' in these structures.

Pain has been considered to be a specific sensation provoked by a sensory input such as intense pressure that is at least potentially damaging to tissue. This view is reflected in the title of the classic work of Hardy, Wolff and Goodell, "Pain Sensations and Reactions" (see suggestions for further reading), and implies that there are physio-- logical mechanisms committed to carrying information specifically about pain. These would include 'pain' receptors in the skin, deep tissue and viscera, 'pain' fibres in the peripheral nervous system that carry the information to specific 'pain' cells in the spinal cord that, in turn, relay information via a specific tract in the cord to the higher structures of the central nervous system. There is no doubt as to the existence of receptors and spinal cord cells that only respond to mechanical or thermal stimuli at intensities that would be expected to provoke pain perception. But the pioneers in pain research, Melzack and Wall, (see suggestions for further reading) distinguish between what they term 'physiological specialisation' and 'psychological specificity'. They point out that a receptor in the skin or nerve fibre might be tuned to respond optimally to a stimulus of a particular nature or intensity but that this does not imply a strict identification between that nerve fibre's activity and a complex perception. The pain theory of Melzack and Wall, albeit highly controversial, has been influential and it is now customary to use the more conservative term 'nociception' (from the latin 'nocere', to hurt), rather than 'pain', when referring to activity in the peripheral nerve and central nervous system.

The axons, or fibres, of the peripheral nervous system have been classified into three groups, labeled A, B, and C fibres. The A fibres are further subdivided into A-alpha, A-beta, A-gamma and A-delta. It is the A-beta, A-delta and the C fibres that are involved in the sensory reaction to touch, pressure and thermal stimulation. There are differences in the rate at which the fibre groups conduct information from peripheral receptors to the spinal cord. A-beta fibres conduct faster than the A-delta and C fibres and are activated by light pressure to the skin. In the A-delta group there are fibres that respond only to high intensity mechanical stimulation. C fibres tend to respond to high intensity mechanical stimulation as well as thermal and chemical stimuli and are the slowest of the groups in conduction rate. In the light of their response characteristics, it might seem reasonable to designate the A-delta and C-fibres as 'pain' fibres, with their predisposition to respond to high intensity mechanical or thermal input. Further, the A-delta fibres could be thought to mediate the first fast phase of pain with the C fibre system being responsible for the later aching phase. But, as the result of investigation of what happens to peripheral fibre input within the spinal cord, such a 'specific' pain designation has been queried (Melzack and Wall, 1991).

The core of the spinal cord is by no means homogeneous but consists of a number of layers or laminae. Concentrated close to the surface, there are cells that are activated predominantly by A-delta and C fibres and respond only to high intensity stimulation. Again, this would seem to constitute evidence for the existence of a 'specific' nociceptive system. But the situation is in fact rather more complicated. A-delta and A-beta fibres project into the deeper layers of the spinal cord and can converge on the same spinal cord cell. These cells will of course respond to mechanical stimulation of high as well as low intensities. Output from both the superficial and deeper located cells is transmitted by way of tracts in the spinal cord to central areas in the brain. Some of these areas are associated with sensory discrimination, but others with arousal and emotion. Input from the cutaneous tissue, muscle or viscera is processed in a similar way in the spinal cord, except that the viscera activate cells in the superficial and deeper layers that also receive cutaneous input. There seem to be no cells in the spinal cord that are activated solely by visceral input. This could explain why pain originating from the viscera, such as the kidney, is often 'referred' to a peripheral body site such as the lower back.

There is also a group of very small cells in the spinal cord that respond to A or C fibre input but which project only locally within the spinal cord. They modulate the activity of the spinal cord neurons that project to the spinal cord tracts, rather than transmit information to central brain structures. Activation of these 'local' cells, or 'inter-neurons', can result in excitation or inhibition of the transmission cells, and they provide a mechanism by which non-nociceptive and nociceptive inputs can be balanced against each other even at this early stage of processing. Cells in the spinal cord not only project to structures in the brainstem and cerebral hemispheres, but are also under the influence of input coming from the higher brain centres, particularly in the brainstem. This control is usually inhibitory and is mediated by the small local interneurons. In addition, the cells in the superficial layers of the spinal cord are under a central inhibitory control which seems to be triggered by the sensory stimulation, while the central control over the cells in the deeper layers of the cord is of a tonic or ongoing nature.

The interactions between central control processes and peripheral inputs are dependent on a range of chemicals found in the central nervous system. These include serotonin, noradrenalin and members of a group of substances known as the endorphins and enkephalins, which affect the nervous system in a manner similar to that of the opiates such as morphine. That these chemicals are involved in nociceptive modulatory processes could be particularly relevant to female pain perception, since there is some evidence (reviewed by Goolkasian, 1985) that reproductory hormones such as estrogen may influence serotonin and noradrenalin production.

This is a lengthy but none-the-less simplified description of the nociceptive mechanisms in the spinal cord. It is however, one which makes apparent how differences can arise in the interpretation of research into the physiology of pain. Some eminent pain researchers promote as the basic nociceptive system the more superficial group of cells in the spinal cord that are activated only by high intensity A-delta and C fibre input. Others have championed the group in the deeper layers of the spinal cord. A compromise position is to accept that both systems are involved, contributing to different aspects of a pain perception. It has been suggested, for example, that the two systems are differentially activated by short lasting or intermittent pain, as compared with continuous or chronic pain. However, there is a general agreement, not only that the spinal cord cells involved in processing nociceptive input are influenced by non-noxious sensory stimulation, but also that they are affected by activity from central brain areas (Liebeskind and Paul, 1977).

The complexity of the nociceptive mechanisms in the spinal cord needs to be borne in mind when interpreting behavioral studies of pain. It is reasonable to expect that noxious inputs are differentially processed by spinal cord cells if they differ in temporal characteristics, for example noxious inputs associated with short-lived experimental pain compared with those emanating from chronic disease such as arthritis which provoke long lasting pain. Variations in the nature and locus of the pain stimulus will also result in different patterns of activity in the A-beta, A-delta and C fibre groups and consequently different patterns of activity in the superficial and deeper spinal nociceptive systems. In addition, control of spinal cord nociceptive mechanisms by higher order brain structures implicates experiential and emotional factors in the perception of pain. This makes the analysis of pain perception in terms of sensory and reactive (ie. 'psychological') subdivisions somewhat questionable. Sex differences in general pain experience, cultural attitudes to pain which are gender related, or differences in interpreting the significance of pain, could influence even the earliest stages of processing of nociceptive information.

In summary, the present physiological evidence indicates that it is an over-simplification to divide sensory input into 'non-painful' and 'painful' categories. Nociceptive processes in the spinal cord depend not only on inputs from sensory events which are potentially tissue damaging, but also on any associated non-noxious stimulation. It is the relationship between sensory inputs that is of importance for pain perception. In the spinal cord the effects of peripheral inputs are also modified by control from brain structures concerned with arousal, emotive and cognitive processes. Consequently, fundamental differences in pain perception between females and males could derive from experiential or attitudinal factors being expressed by way of these modulating influences. Further, since the central control over the spinal cord cells involve chemicals that can be affected by female reproductive hormones, constitutionally-based sex differences in pain perception are also a possibility.

SEX DIFFERENCES IN RESPONSE TO EXPERIMENTAL PAIN

Experimental studies of pain perception indicate that women may be more sensitive to pain than men. A consistent finding in a number of studies carried out at Stirling

University is a distinctive difference in pain thresholds between male and female students. In our studies, pain is produced by placing a blunt metal rod (pain algometer) on the sternum (breast bone) and slowly increasing the pressure until pain is reported. This pressure value is taken as the pain 'threshold'. Women appear to be more sensitive to pain, reporting pain at lower pressure values than male subjects.

Our results agree with those of previous studies which have used a variety of stimuli to evoke pain including heat, cold, electrical and a variety of mechanical stimuli. Body sites have included the forehead, inner surface of the arm, fingers, and achilles tendon and the upper lip. In a highly systematic study by Fischer (1987), pain thresholds to mechanical pressure were measured on the surface of nine different muscles. Except for one, the gluteus medius muscle (inner aspect of the lower back), the pain threshold of the female subjects was significantly lower than that of the males. However, for every study that has reported an increased pain sensitivity in women, there is also one recording no difference. For example, no differences in pain sensitivity were reported in the pioneering work of Hardy, Wolff and Goodell (1967).

To complicate matters further, differences in pain tolerance have been reported where no differences in threshold appear. In general, studies of pain tolerance are more consistent in finding sex differences; women are less tolerant of pain than men (see Goolkasian, 1985, for a review of the literature). It has been claimed that pain tolerance is more sensitive to 'psychological' factors than pain threshold, which is regarded as more a product of basic sensory factors (Liebeskind and Paul, 1977). We have argued earlier in this review against making such distinctions in pain perception; what these data might be revealing is a difference in pain perception between males and females that is more obvious when the intensity of noxious stimulation is clearly in the painful range. Sex differences in pain perception may be only minimally affected by the tendency of women, as compared to men, to report a weak stimulus as painful (ie. threshold effects). Instead, females may be markedly more sensitive to actual pain experience (ie. to supra-threshold effects; levels of noxious stimulation which will be experienced by all subjects, both male and female, as definitely painful) perceiving this supra-threshold stimulation as more intense or distressing than males and thus being less willing to tolerate it.

It is not clear why sex differences only emerge from some studies of pain thresholds. Comparisons among studies are difficult to make because the procedures adopted vary widely. For example, in the 'cold pressor' test of pain sensitivity the subject's arm is immersed in cold water and the pain develops over a longer duration than the pain resulting from the use of a pain algometer. Different tests involve the use of various forms of stimuli, presented for varying periods of temporal exposure. These differences could be associated with the different types of control exerted by central brain structures at the level of the spinal cord. Perhaps, if researchers into experimental pain were to adopt more than one form of noxious stimulation in their studies, the reviewer could be more confident in the general reliablity of their results.

In a suprathreshold situation, if female subjects are asked to rate the intensity of an experimentally induced thermal pain either by using a linear scale, or by matching its intensity to the brightness of a light, they tend to rate the pain as being of a higher intensity than that reported by male subjects for stimuli of equivalent intensity (Feine *et al.*, 1991). These researchers also provide evidence based on the use of similar scales, that women are more sensitive than men in discriminating between noxious heat stimuli that are above threshold.

It has been claimed that sex differences between subject and investigator influence pain ratings, with men tending to register lower pain ratings to a female experimenter and women tending to report higher pain ratings to a male experimenter (Levine and De Simone, 1991). Similar cross-sex effects have been observed for threshold studies, but as with much else in the field of study of experimental pain, such effects are not reported consistently. Even when present, these kinds of effects cannot be taken as evidence for unreliable reporting on the part of the subjects. Instead, they may be regarded as exemplifying the effects of situational factors on pain perception. The gender of the experimenter is one such situational factor. Other situational factors involving the context of an injury – on the sports field rather than in a car crash; the meaning of the pain – life giving as in childbirth, compared with life threatening as in a heart attack, are also likely to affect the perception of the pain involved.

One explanation for the apparent sex differences in pain threshold is that in experimental situations women are more willing than men to label a 'sensation' as painful. Goolkasian (1985) has argued that in many reports of an heightened pain sensitivity in women, there is confusion between the subject's ability to discriminate between a painful and non-painful stimulus and their criteria for labeling a stimulus as painful. Goolkasian uses a particular form of psychophysical procedure, derived from signal detection theory, to study pain thresholds. In her tests, subjects are randomly exposed using a large number of trials to thermal stimuli of three different intensities. They are asked to label their perceptual responses using six different categories, 'nothing', 'warm', 'hot', 'faintly painful', 'moderately painful' and 'strongly painful'. She then uses a special form of mathematical analysis that, it is claimed, can distinguish variations in the ability to discriminate a stimulus as painful from changes in criteria for reporting a stimulus as being painful. While she reports that men and women can differ in their pain sensitivities to thermal stimulation, she found no difference in their willingness to label a stimulus as painful. Her data, then, offer no support to the interpretation that sex differences reported in other studies represent biases in labeling rather than differences in discrimination.

The use of such rigorous psychophysical techiques is exemplary. Nevertheless, it is important to emphasize again that what is known of the complex interactive nature of the physiological mechanisms mediating pain, makes distinction between 'sensory' and 'judgemental' elements of pain perception difficult.

PAIN AND HORMONAL FLUCTUATIONS

A number of investigators have shown that the sensitivity of women to pain varies over the menstrual cycle. Goolkasian (1985) reported an increase in supra-threshold pain sensitivity fifteen to twenty one days into the cycle, corresponding to the ovulatory phase. This increase was not attributable to criteria biases. It was not evident in women using oral contraceptives. She found no cyclical changes in the ability to discriminate between non-noxious thermal stimuli of different intensities but found women, during the ovulatory phase, to be significantly more sensitive to differences between noxious and non-noxious thermal stimulation. There is now reasonably good agreement that women show an increase in pain sensitivity in the middle of the menstrual cycle. Indeed some of the previously cited confusion in the fields of sex differences in the perception of experimental pain could stem from failures to monitor the menstrual status of female subjects.

The mechanisms by which female sex hormones modify sensitivity to pain are unclear. Neurochemicals related to nociceptive modulation are likely to be involved. It has been suggested by Goolkasian and others, that the preovulatory increase in estrogen levels results in a decrease in the catabolism of serotonin, which is one of the chemicals implicated in the inhibitory control over spinal cord cells. Interaction between reproductive hormones and the brain's natural opiates could also explain changes in pain sensitivity over the menstrual cycle, but there is no evidence for such an interaction as yet.

Goolkasian (1985) has also reported that women who experience pain during menstruation ('dysmenorrhoea') fail to show a cyclical change in pain sensitivity; in such women sensitivity remains relatively high throughout the month. A hormone called 'prostaglandin' is implicated in dysmenorrhoea, promoting cramping of the uterus. Prostaglandin does not provoke pain itself but sensitizes sensory receptors to noxious stimulation. If it is higher in dysmenorrhoeic women throughout the menstrual cycle, this mechanism could account for their more uniform pain responsitivity. However, not all studies of dysmenorrhoeic women find an heightened sensitivity to pain. Discrepancies in results could reflect differences in the criteria used to classify subjects as dysmenorrhoeic, whether, for example, by pain intensity in a representative sample of healthy women, or by specialist clinic attendance. In addition, the extent to which some dysmenorrhoeic women are successful in adapting to, or coping with, menstrual pain, could be associated with benign changes in their attitudes to noxious episodes which might counter any sensitization of peripheral nociceptive processes by prostaglandin.

Studies of pain sensitivity during the menstrual cycle provide useful clues as to what might underlie differences in pain sensitivity between women and men. They demonstrate that a range of factors could be implicated. The variation in pain sensitivity with varying levels of female sex hormones indicate that sex hormones affect, even if indirectly, nociceptive mechanisms in women. Differences in the sensitivity cycles of dysmenorrhoeic and non-dysmenorrhoeic women possibly reflect the influence of prostaglandin on the earliest stages of nociception in some women. On the other hand, research on the pain perception of dysmenorrheic women opens up the question as to the role that previous pain experience may have in making judgements about novel noxious events.

A general conclusion that can be drawn from the studies that have compared the perception by females and males of experimental pain, is that there are no reports of male subjects showing higher pain sensitivity than females whether judged in terms of threshold, tolerance, discrimination ability or pain intensity ratings. However, a significant number of studies have found the opposite to be true. Whether this is due to differences between the sexes in basic physiology or complex psychological processes has not been determined and arguably, from a neuropsychological perspective, it would be hard to do so.

SEX DIFFERENCES IN PAIN INCIDENCE

There is good evidence that girls experience more incidences of pain than boys. They report experiencing abdominal pain, headache, and 'growing' pains more frequently than boys, as well as suffering more often from musculoskeletal pain associated with juvenile rheumatoid arthritis. However, the picture for adults is far less clear. Epidemological studies show that women make more use of medical services than men and have a higher sickness or morbidity rate than men (see Chapter 1). It is not surprising then that a number of national surveys using epidemiological methodology have revealed that women also report more instances of pain. In a study based on a survey of Canadian households Crook *et al.* (1984) reported a higher incidence of episodic pain in women related either to head and face, abdomen and chest, or lower extremities (8.5 percent of the total population as compared with 3.6 percent incidence in males). A tendancy to a higher incidence of persistent pain was also reported for women (14.5 percent versus 12.6 percent). Similar results have been reported from New Zealand, the United States and Wales (James *et al.*, 1991; Von Korff *et al.*, 1988; Waters, 1970). The difference between the sexes in these studies was mainly in abdominal and headache pain and not in joint, back or chest pain. A higher prevalence of urogenital pain was also found among women, and up to thirty percent of women reported pain associated with menstruation (see Chapter 2 for discussion of related aspects of menstruation). However, with respect to pains that are common to men and women, there is little evidence that there is any difference in the reported levels of pain. An interpretation of these data is that women are more sensitive to noxious input involving the head and abdomen. Since they do not report more pain than men for musculoskeletal problems, this bias is not the result of an enhanced willingness to label somatic symptoms as painful.

There are, however, difficulties in interpreting epidemological data on sex differences in pain incidence. Women appear to suffer more incidences of pain than men but this may be the direct or indirect result of constitutional differences relating to menstruation. Headache and abdominal pain can be associated with menstruation and headache with the use of oral contraception. Unfortunately, not all of the investigators of clinical pain incidence, including those looking specifically at headache, have determined to what extent headache and abdominal pains reported by women were related to the menstrual cycle or the use of oral contraceptives.

It is also possible that regular experience of discomforture during the menstrual cycle sensitizes the nociceptive mechanisms subserving head and abdominal regions. Further, it should be remembered that spinal cells that are activated by inputs from the viscera also receive excitatory cutaneous and muscle input and this convergence may exacerbate any predisposition for women to experience abdominal discomforture.

Whatever the reason for sex differences in pain histories, we might expect this difference to be significant in determining the nature of female pain responsivity. Pain experience, of a non-traumatic nature, could provide a natural training opportunity to refine the ability to label and distinguish between noxious stimuli of varying intensity. This would result in women possessing an enhanced sensitivity to noxious stimulation as well the capacity to discriminate between noxious stimuli of different intensities.

WOMEN AND THE EXPERIENCE OF CHILDBIRTH PAIN

A major pain experience unique to women is that accompanying childbirth. Not all women report pain during labor, particularly after the first birth. However, for many, the pain is the worst they will ever experience. In the initial stages of birth, the pain is highly correlated with each contraction and probably results from the dilation of the cervix and, to a certain extent, the activity of uterine muscle (Bonica, 1984). Pain is usually described as increasing in intensity during the first stage of labor as the cervix increases in dilation. First stage contraction pain is most often located in the lower abdomen but quite commonly is perceived as emanating from the upper abdomen or back. It may be accompanied by continuous back pain. It reaches a peak at the end of the first stage and during the second stage of birth as the fetus passes into the birth canal, stretching, and possibly damaging, the structures of the vagina and perineum. Pain can also arise from pressure on other pelvic structures such as the urethra and rectum.

Labor pain is often regarded as something of a puzzle since it accompanies a natural body function and is present even during normal healthy births. Accordingly, such pain is sometimes considered to reflect inadequate preparation for the birth, the adoption of inappropriate positions during labor, over-reaction to stress and so forth (Eysenck, 1961; Dick Read, 1942; Kitzinger, 1962). Others have speculated that it is solely due to the medicalization of childbirth, prevalent within Western society but this contention cannot be supported since labor pain is reported by women in all societies (Melzack, 1984), and births which are free of any medical intervention, as well as those which are highly medicalized, can be associated with high levels of pain (Kitzinger, 1989).

One explanation for labor pain is that it is the consequence of the human upright posture leading to a narrow and particularly complex pelvic structure. Given the large size of the highly evolved human brain and the narrowness of the human pelvis, the passage of the baby's head through the pelvis is likely to be a 'tight squeeze'. This will give rise to noxious stimulation and consequentially, pain. Any anatomical mismatch between the size of the baby's head and the mother's birth canal could thus exacerbate pain during the second stage of labor. It is difficult, however, to explain the considerable pain of early labor, when the fetus has yet to enter the birth canal, by reference to complications in pelvic anatomy.

Around two thirds of normal human births occur at night. Most diurnal mammals show a similar birthing pattern. However, human births accompanied by complications tend to occur during the day. The existence of this diurnal pattern emphasizes that even in humans giving birth is under a complex endocrine control involving a delicate balance between a number of factors which prepare the uterus, cervix and muscles of the birth canal for an orderly sequence of contraction, dilation and expulsion. The nociceptive elements of childbirth could be in part the consequence of this balance being, for some reason, less than optimal. This speculation is supported by the observation that normal healthy births occurring during the day, against an apparent natural trend, are reported as being more painful and stressful than night births (Harkness and Gijsbers, 1989).

Whatever the organic reasons for labor pain, there has been considerable interest in the possible role of psychosocial factors These include social class, attitudes towards the baby, anxiety and personality characteristics, prepared childbirth training, and the presence of the woman's partner during labor. Melzack and colleagues working in Canada, for example, have found significant associations between young maternal age, low social class and high levels of pain (see Melzack, 1984). However, a Scottish study (Niven and Gijsbers, 1984) found no significant correlations between these factors. This may have been due to differences in the populations studied; Melzack's subjects were drawn from a big city (Montreal), whereas ours were from a more mixed rural and urban community where the extremes of poverty and privilege are less apparent.

The desirability of pregnancy has generally been found to correlate negatively with labor pain (eg. Eysenck, 1961; Niven and Gijsbers, 1984). However Astbury (1980), who assessed desirability in the third trimester when negative attitudes towards the baby are generally more stable, found no relationship between unplanned pregnancy or negative attitudes towards the baby and subsequent levels of pain in childbirth.

Studies which have examined the relationship between personality factors and the experience of pain in childbirth have reported inconsistent findings. Eysenck (1961) in an English study found that subjects who scored highly on a measure of 'extraversion', reported higher levels of labor pain than those scoring more highly on a measure of 'introversion'. Reading and Cox (1985) found that subjects assessed as 'neurotic' on the EPI had higher levels of labor pain and attributed this to the higher levels of arousal and anxiety which neurotic subjects would be postulated to have during childbirth. In comparison, Scott-Palmar and Skevington (1981) found neuroticism to be related to lower levels of labor pain. Astbury (1980) found no relationship between trait anxiety and levels of labor pain. The reasons for these inconsistencies are partly methodological. The timing of the assessments of personality varied between studies and the meaning that they had for the subjects may have markedly affected the results obtained. The inconsistent findings may also be due to the fact that women in childbirth do not necessarily demonstrate their 'normal personality'. "The cowardly can be un-expectedly brave, the strong surprisingly weak, the out-going unusually quiet and the polite devastatingly rude. The demands of giving birth are exceptional and they bring out exceptional characteristics in those who go through it" (Niven, 1992, p. 52).

Similarly, research findings have yet to establish conclusively that participation in ante-natal or prepared childbirth training (PCT) has positive effects on pain in labor (Ante-natal training is the term used in the UK, PCT, the term used in the US). Many of the studies published in this area have methodological problems which prevent us drawing firm conclusions about their effectiveness. A few studies have attempted to allocate class attendance on a random basis so that attenders and non-attenders would be matched for socioeconomic status, age, parity etc. However, drop out rates varied between classes so that at the end of the study, the inequalities were still evident. Despite these difficulties some consistency of outcome is found, in that class attenders report increased maternal satisfaction with childbirth and decreased use of analgesics.

Reduced analgesic use during childbirth may be due to the reassuring effects of class attendance; to the use of psychoprophalactic techniques such as relaxation and breathing exercises which are designed to reduce pain and which are taught in classes; or to information conveyed about obstetric analgesics in these classes which sometimes tends to discourage their use (Melzack, 1984). In his Canadian studies, Melzack has found that women who had attended PCT classes had significantly lower levels of labor pain compared with those who had not gone to these classes. Though the vast majority of his subjects (PCT and non-PCT) used epidural anaesthesia, women who had attended classes tended to use it later in labor, especially when their

PCT educator had strongly encouraged her students to forgo it (Melzack, 1984). Thus, it seems that his PCT subjects did generally have lower levels of labor pain. However, the intensity of their pain was such that, though they deferred accepting an epidural, they eventually sought to relieve their pain in this way, despite in some cases having been 'warned off' its use. Therefore, although PCT appeared to be related to lower levels of labor pain in this study, it was not related to *painless* childbirth. In our Scottish study, we found that women who had attended antenatal classes in their current pregnancy had lower levels of pain recorded during the active phase of the first stage of labor, even when the effects of age, socioeconomic status, and more positive expectations of birth were statistically controlled. These results would indicate that antenatal education was effective in reducing labor pain and that this effect was not solely due to the relationship between class attendance and variables which independently affected obstetric outcome or pain levels (Niven, 1986; Niven and Gijsbers, 1984).

Thus, although the results of research are not conclusive, there is evidence that a number of psychological factors can modulate the experience of labor pain. Other factors, such as the presence of a partner can be positive or negative depending on the context. Melzack (1984) in Canada, found that women report more intense labor pain when their husbands are present than when they are absent. A general analysis of the relationship between labor pain levels and the presence of the woman's partner or other chosen birth companion carried out on Scottish subjects (Niven, 1985), found no significant differences in pain levels between the women who had their partners with them, and those who did not. However, when the parturant's assessment of his presence was taken into consideration, women who positively welcomed his presence had lower levels of labor pain when compared with all other subjects. This finding suggests that it is not the partner's presence *per se* that is important but the laboring woman's feelings about his presence.

Lists of parameters that can be significantly correlated with the intensity of labor pain can be compiled. However, at this stage of our understanding of labor pain, it is more worthwhile to address the question as to why such factors affect the pain. For example, women who have had an experience of intense pain, outwith childbirth, report lower levels of childbirth pain than parturants who have only experienced mild pain (Niven, in press). Evidence from this study indicates that the experience of significant pain can promote the development of a repertoire of pain coping strategies, providing the experience is not overwhelmingly stressful. These include strategies based on relaxation, distraction, imagery and normalization of the pain. Some of these strategies can be marshalled to cope with the pain of childbirth and their successful application during labor is thus associated with lower labor pain levels.

However, it should be emphasized that the relationship between previous pain experience and labor pain is not straightforward. About one out of ten women in the population studied claimed that they had experienced little or no pain outwith childbirth. These women reported the lowest levels of labor pain and perhaps represented a special group with particularly low nociceptive sensitivity (Niven and Gijsbers, 1989). In addition, it is likely that the successful transfer of pain coping strategies to the labor situation will be affected by a range of factors such as the social and physical environment in which the birth is taking place, the rate of development of the pain and the fatigue of the parturient.

There is conflicting evidence as to whether the sense of being in control during childbirth is related to lower levels of labor pain. Low (1989) has identified confidence in being able to handle the pain as being an important predictor of childbirth pain. It is possible that confidence in this regard is related to the experience of successfully coping with pain in previous situations and anticipating being able to cope during labor. Women who have experienced intense pain previous to childbirth might not only be better equipped to handle the intense pain of childbirth but may also be relatively confident of their capacity to do so. Arguably, analysis of the use of coping strategies during childbirth is central to understanding the role of psychosocial factors in labor pain.

COPING WITH PAIN

Most people, to a greater or lesser degree, have developed a repertoire of strategies to handle painful episodes. If women suffer more episodes of pain than men, the question arises as to whether there are sex differences in pain coping styles. Most studies of styles of coping with pain have focussed on chronic pain, usually back pain. Several coping questionnaires have been developed which include systematically compiled lists of strategies in common use. However, while there is considerable documentation on the deployment of various strategies by the chronic pain patient, evidence for their efficacy is less substantial. This is not altogether surprising since chronic pain is, by definition, persistent. Consequently, a particular strategy might be modifying the quantity or quality of a persistent pain, but this would be hard to confirm. There appears to be little evidence for differences between males and females in coping with chronic pain. Studies of how people deal with episodic or acute pain might give better insight into the development and use of pain strategies. Accordingly, it might prove instructive to question subjects who participate in studies of experimental pain whether they are spontaneously employing some form of mental coping strategy.

The argument that advantages can be derived from a certain amount of pain experience assumes that the strategies acquired are of a positive and not of a negative or 'catastrophising' nature. In addition, any cognitive advantage that experiencing pain might grant would also have to be balanced against any sensitization of basic nociceptive processes which would be disadvantageous. For example, we have found the experience of high levels of menstrual pain to be associated with lower levels of labor pain, possibly because the intensely painful menstrual experience promotes strategy development (Niven, 1986). But Melzack and his colleagues, in a number of studies concerned with labor pain, find that pain associated with menstruation is positively correlated overall with labor pain (eg. Melzack, 1984). This positive relationship is thought to reflect an enhanced tendency in some women to secrete prostaglandin. This would result in increased strength of uterine contractions as well as enhanced periperal nociception both during menstruation and childbirth. The difference between our obervations and those of Melzack may lie in relative cognitive advantages arising from pain experience and the disadvantages stemming from the sensitization of peripheral nociceptive processes.

Berlinger *et al.* (1989) have also studied pain arising from medical abortion in the early part of pregnancy. They reported moderate levels of pain could be associated with the procedures of suction-curettage that were used. As with the pain of childbirth, there was a large individual variation. An emotional factor, pre-abortion depression, was found to be significantly related to the pain, as was a history of dysmenorrhea. This suggests that in abortion pain, attitudes might be as important as any predisposition to peripheral nociception.

Studies of pain relating to childbirth have been particularly fruitful in providing an insight into how women cope with pain. They also illustrate how pain perception is composed of highly interactive emotional, cognitive, as well as sensory components. If from childhood, women are predisposed to experience more episodes of pain than men, they may also have greater reason and opportunity to aquire a sophisticated repertoire of strategies for dealing with pain. The utilization of this repertoire would not only differentiate their pain perception from that of men, but would also be of particular benefit in potentially painful situations specific to women such as childbirth.

WOMEN AND 'SYNDROME' PAIN

Our previous discussion has suggested that women are especially competent in making judgements concerning pain and in coping with naturally occurring painful experiences such as menstruation and childbirth. These conclusions may be at odds with the observation that women are vastly more likely to be diagnosed as suffering from a number of painful syndromes that have been thought to be psychosomatic or psychogenic in origin. These include Fibromyalgia, characterized by a pervasive muscloskeletal pain and muscle tenderness; Irritable Bowel Syndrome (IBS) a gastrointestinal disorder accompanied by pain in the abdomen; Repetition Strain Injury (RSI), which is mainly expressed as pain in the upper limbs, trunk and neck; and Atypical Facial Pain. The reported ratios of women to men complaining of these symptoms vary from three to one for IBS (Ford, 1986), up to about eight to one for Fibromyalgia (Felson, 1989). Since it has been difficult to identify any definite organic disorder in subjects presenting with these pains, they are sometimes considered, by default, as being of psychological origin. The implication is that women are prone to interpreting non-noxious stimuli as painful, ie. that they are not competent in making judgements concerning pain or, alternatively, do not cope effectively with the pain that they experience.

However, it must be emphasized that the diagnosis of these syndromes as psychosomatic is by default. Psychological disturbances have sometimes been found in association with these types of pain, but since the pain is often persistent and disabling, it is not altogether surprising that some subjects show symptoms of stress, or of depression which is generally now held to be a *consequence* of chronic pain rather than a *cause* (Feinmann, 1985). Mild depression is more likely to be found in association with chronic pain in women as compared with men (Magni *et al.*, 1990). This might be because depression is more common in women than men (see Chapter 9) or be a reflection of women's recognition of their failure to cope successfully with an enduring pain.

Repetition strain injury (RSI) pain, as the term implies, is experienced by people involved in tasks demanding repeated fast manual movement such as working at a keyboard. The sex difference in reporting this type of pain probably arises because tasks of this nature are mainly carried out by women. Since RSI is a job related pain, failure to make a clear cut organic diagnosis can be particularly contentious if compensation or absence from work is involved. There is evidence that, despite RSI's clear cut ergonomic dependence, the medical profession can be less than sympathetic to women who report symptoms of this syndrome: The title of an Australian study by Reid, Ewan and Lowy (1991), *Pilgrimage of pain: the illness experiences of women with repetition strain injury and the search for credibility* highlights their problem. Difficulties may however also arise when a patient suffering syndrome pain encounters a sympathetic medical practitioner who may resort to unnecessary treatment in search for cure. For example, women suffering from IBS may undergo a series of unsuccessful abdominal operations (Chaudhary and Truelove, 1962).

WOMEN AND COMPETENCE IN PAIN PERCEPTION

Pain, like illness, can be disruptive of normal patterns of daily activity. But its necessary role in healthy living cannot be denied. This is reflected in the extensive dedication of physiological mechanisms to the process of transforming peripheral nociceptive information into an appropriate perception of pain. Never-the-less, most of us adopt life styles designed to minimize pain experience. There are however, exceptions. Competitive athletes often use pain as a measure of their training efficacy, as do professional dancers. While there are reports of decreased pain sensitivity as well as increased pain tolerance in athletes (Scott and Gijsbers, 1981), for pain to be of use in training, athletes must maintain the capacity to discriminate between relatively benign pain and pain related to a potentially incapacitating injury. There is reason to believe that athletes are also particularly competent in using pain coping strategies appropriate to the particular characteristics of the sport. Strategies leading to the diminution of pain perception may be appropriate to contact sports, but would be inappropriate to a sport such as squash where pain that signals tendon strain is probable.

We suggest that women, like competitive athletes, develop a high level of competence in dealing with nociceptive information. There is good evidence from the experimental study of pain that hormonal factors sensitize nociceptive processes in women, and females from an early age report noxious stimulation as being more intense or unpleasant than do males. Females also from an early age tend to differ from males in their everyday experience of episodic pain and markedly so as adults with the onset of menstruation and the experience of childbirth. From what we know of the neural mechanisms mediating pain, its perception is dependent to a considerable extent on cognitive and emotional processes that are going to be shaped by experimental factors. Consequently, it is to be expected that these constitutional and experimental differences will combine to produce distinct differences between men and women in their pain perception. This could lead to the conclusion that females are indeed the 'suffering' sex. Although the negative consequences of failure to cope with pain are not to be discounted, a positive view of differences in pain sensitivity between the sexes is that women possess an enhanced perceptual competence that is adapted to their specific nociceptive experience related to childbearing and nurturing.

FURTHER READING

Hardy, J.D., Wolff, H.G. and Goodell, H. (1967). *Pain sensations and reactions*. New York: Hafner Publishing Co.

Melzack, R. and Wall, P. (1991). *The challenge of pain*. New York: Penguin Books.

Niven, C. (1992). *Psychological care for families: Before, during and after birth*. Oxford: Butterworth Heinemann.

5

CARDIOVASCULAR HEALTH AND DISEASE IN WOMEN

KATHLEEN A. LIGHT AND SUSAN S. GIRDLER

CB#7175 Medical Research Building A, Department of Psychiatry, University of North Carolina at Chapel Hill, Chapel Hill, North Carolina 27599-7175, USA

INTRODUCTION

Cardiovascular disease is the number one cause of death in industrialized nations, for women as well as for men. Yet women, especially younger women, show a lower incidence of cardiac-related death than men of the same age. The primary intent of this chapter is to explore possible reasons for the relatively 'protected' status of women compared to men with regard to coronary heart disease and its major disease precursors, hypertension and atherosclerotic vascular disease. However, the secondary intent is to underscore the opposite side of this coin. Despite the advantages associated with being female, no other disorder causes as much premature disability and death in women as cardiovascular disease and thus clinical treatment and research to reduce this excess mortality should be pursued with the same urgency as for men.

EPIDEMIOLOGY OF CARDIOVASCULAR DISEASE IN MEN AND WOMEN

As long ago as 1768, William Heberden observed in his book, *Commentaries on the History and Cure of Diseases*, that the disorder of heart-related chest pain (angina pectoris) was far more prevalent in men than women (Higgins, 1990). Over the next 200 years, this perception that coronary heart disease was primarily a problem of middle-aged and older men became part of accepted medical dogma. As a result, many of the major epidemiological studies designed to identify factors which increase or decrease risk of this disorder have not included women as participants or have underrepresented women, particularly those over the age of 65, the critical age range. This has led in part to less understanding about the factors influencing the development of heart disease in women as compared to men.

Nevertheless, recent epidemiological findings have made it clear that, although this disorder affects women on an average of a decade later in life than men, coronary heart disease is the leading cause of death in women just as in men. In the United States, where roughly 550,000 people die each year from heart disease, approximately 250,000 are female (Eaker *et al.*, 1987). However, in younger age groups, women do appear somewhat protected from this lethal disorder. Of the nearly 100,000 deaths annually in individuals under 65 years of age, over 70,000 are in men, resulting in a ratio of almost three male deaths for every female death from coronary causes. In contrast, among persons older than 65 years, deaths due to heart disease in women actually slightly exceed those in men, with both genders averaging over 200,000 deaths annually (Eaker *et al.*, 1987; Higgins, 1990). Although these numbers are influenced by the fact that more women than men survive into their 70's and 80's and in fact heart disease afflicts a slightly larger percentage of males than females even among the elderly, it is still apparent that the protective effects associated with being female are largely gone by the age of 65. Why would women demonstrate a decreased risk of heart disease relative to men and furthermore, why would this feminine advantage disappear after the age of 65? Firm answers to these questions are not yet clearly documented, but most medical and scientific experts point to the primary proven risk factors for men—serum cholesterol, high blood pressure (hypertension), cigarette smoking, obesity, diabetes, lack of physical activity and behavioral patterns or lifestyles associated with increased psychological stress. The best evidence now available examines gender differences in these risk factors and also emphasizes the importance of the female reproductive hormones, particularly estrogen, which may interact and modulate the effects of each of the traditional risk factors documented for men. Estrogen reduction after the menopause is also thought to be the principal modulator influencing the disappearance of female protection from heart disease after the age of 65.

PHYSICAL FACTORS INFLUENCING CORONARY DISEASE AND HEALTH OUTCOMES IN WOMEN

Blood Pressure

Hypertension or sustained high blood pressure (defined as diastolic pressure $\geqslant$ 90mmHg) is a major risk factor for morbidity and mortality from coronary heart disease and stroke in both men and women (Kannel, 1977; Anastos *et al.*, 1991). Hypertension is presumed to contribute to the development of heart disease both by overworking the heart leading to structural changes in this vital organ and by inducing changes in blood vessels. These vascular changes occur in the structural elements of vessels that are involved in constriction and dilation and also at the fragile inner wall or endothelium of the vessel where damage can increase fat deposition and formation of plaques (atherogenesis). Since hypertension has been well established as a risk factor in many studies, major public health initiatives have been undertaken in many countries to educate people about the health impact of this symptomless disorder, and to attempt to assess the health benefits of treatment to reduce blood pressure in as many hypertensive individuals as possible. As a result, medications to lower blood pressure are currently the most common category of prescriptions written by American physicians (Baum *et al.*, 1988).

Women have lower blood pressure on average and lesser prevalence of hypertension than men from adolescence until approximately the age of 55. Also, when clinically identified as having hypertension, women exceed men in the proportion who successfully control their blood pressure through treatment, possibly because more women than men strictly comply with the recommended treatment regimen. However, when the full age range of the population is considered together, the elderly as well as younger groups, and when persons with controlled as well as uncontrolled hypertension are included, the prevalence of hypertension is equally high in women as in men (Anastos *et al.*, 1991).

Although the major public health initiatives to lower blood pressure have been directed at women as well as men, definitive evidence indicating that such treatment reduces risk of mortality from heart disease among women of all ages is still not available. Of the seven large scale investigations completed to date, only four included women as participants (Anastos *et al.*, 1991). Results of these major research efforts from Australia, the US, the UK and Europe have yielded inconsistent findings. The Australian Therapeutic Trial in Mild Hypertension (Management Committee, 1980, 1981) compared the effects of drug treatment versus placebo, and reported evidence of a significant benefit of treatment for men but not for women when stroke and non-fatal as well as fatal coronary events were considered together. This result is somewhat misleading, for women on treatment actually demonstrated a greater percentage reduction in these events compared to women on placebo than was shown by men on treatment compared to placebo (36 percent for women versus 26 percent for men). Because epidemiologic evidence has documented that untreated women experience these fatal and nonfatal end-points at a substantially lower rate than untreated men, it is necessary to include more women than men in the sample to achieve differences between treatment and placebo conditions which meet standard statistical criteria for significance. In this as most previous investigations, the reverse occurred; twice as many men as women were studied, making it unlikely that a true benefit for treatment could be detected in women.

In the US-sponsored Hypertension Detection and Follow-up Program (HDFP) Cooperative Group (1979) investigation, benefits of stepped-care (involving vigorous efforts to add to or change medication until high blood pressure is fully controlled) were compared with usual care (including antihypertensive drugs but with a less strict focus on lowering to normal pressure levels) in a sample of whom 46 percent were women and 44 percent were black. This study demonstrated a significant reduction in coronary mortality in black women given the stricter stepped-care (28 percent) and smaller but significant reductions in men (19 percent and 15 percent for black and white men). White women, however, showed no benefit of stepped-care versus usual care and, in fact, showed a slight trend in the reverse direction (Schnall *et al.*, 1984). Why would stepped-care have a greater benefit for black versus white women? One contributing factor may be the fact that black women tend to develop hypertension at a younger age than white women and so, in these age-matched samples, the black women had been hypertensive on average for up to 10 years longer and may thus have represented a group with more vascular damage where usual care is more likely to prove insufficient. It has been observed that black women show coronary mortality rates that are twice as great as white women between the ages of 40–60 years. Another contributing factor is that black people in the US have traditionally received less access to health care; for black women, the differences in treatment between stepped and usual care might be greater than for white women, for whom usual care may have approached the same strict standards as stepped care.

In the UK, the Medical Research Council Work Party (1985), reported the results of their Trial of Treatment of Mild Hypertension which compared placebo versus drug treatment in a predominantly white sample of whom 48 percent were women. This study yielded an unexpected significant difference between men and women in the effects of drug treatment. Mortality from all causes was significantly reduced in men (–15 percent) but increased in women (+26 percent) among those on active drugs versus placebo. These results, together with the HDFP observation, suggest that vigorous drug treatment in white women with mild to moderate hypertension may lead to adverse health outcomes in more patients than benefit from such treatment. It is important to underscore that the follow-up intervals in both these studies were relatively short and that most women tested were younger than 65 years of age, after which the prevalence of coronary fatalities accelerates in women. Over a longer time period, and particularly later in the life span, the benefits to women of drug treatment to lower blood pressure are expected to be greater.

The most recent large-scale investigation of the potential benefits of lowering high blood pressure is from the European Working Party on High Blood Pressure in the Elderly (Amery et al., 1985). This investigation was the first to over-represent women to compensate for their lower prevalence of coronary mortality; females constituted 70 percent of the sample. The age at entry was 60 years or older, approximately when women show their acceleration in prevalence of heart disease, and the follow-up interval was relatively long at 12 years. Even though the total sample was much smaller than those of the previously cited investigations, this project was more appropriately designed to compare the benefits of antihypertensive drug treatment versus placebo in older women and men. The findings revealed that elderly women did indeed benefit from drug treatment; women on active drugs showed an 18 percent reduction in mortality from coronary disease and stroke relative to women on placebo. Nevertheless, men demonstrated a much greater benefit, showing a 47 percent reduction in this mortality rate. Thus, evidence indicates that during the latter years of the life-span when deaths from heart disease are higher, women show a significant benefit of drug treatment for hypertension in the form of reduced mortality from cardiovascular disorders, but even during this time period the benefit from treatment for men is roughly 2.5 times greater than for women. At younger ages, the benefit of drug treatment for white women is still doubtful and further study is needed to clarify whether there may even be an adverse effect of treatment for these women.

Serum Cholesterol and Lipoproteins

High levels of total cholesterol in the blood (>240 mg/dl) are associated with increased risk of death from heart disease in both men and women in those countries where coronary heart disease is a major cause of death. Blood cholesterol levels increase with age in women up to the age of 65 and then a slight decline in cholesterol has been observed. Cholesterol is implicated in the development of heart disease because of its postulated role in enhancing atherogenesis, where the inner walls of blood vessels (including those supplying the working muscles of the heart) develop first fatty streaks and later raised lesions which can grow until they fill most of or all of the vessel opening, creating an obstruction compromising the blood supply to the surrounding tissue.

Although total cholesterol has been shown to be a good predictor of the risk of heart disease, more specific blood lipid measures have been shown to be better predictors. High levels of low density lipoprotein cholesterol (LDL-C) increase risk of coronary disease, while high levels of high density lipoprotein cholesterol (HDL-C) decrease such risk. As a way of combining these two factors, one increasing and one decreasing risk, the HDL-C/LDL-C ratio or the ratio of total cholesterol divided by HDL-C have also been used and proven to be associated with lower risk of coronary morbidity and mortality (Eaker *et al.*, 1987; Lipid Metabolism Branch, 1980).

During their reproductive years, women develop atherogenic changes in their coronary arteries at a slower rate than men. Young women have more extensive fatty streaks in their vessels than men of the same age, corresponding perhaps to their greater overall body fat to total body weight ratio. By early middle age, however, a larger proportion of fatty streaks have progressed to raised lesions in men than in women and further progression to partial or total occlusion of coronary arteries also continues more rapidly in men (McGill and Stern, 1979). One explanation for this slower rate of atherogenic change in women which has been suggested is that women have higher levels of HDL-C and lower total cholesterol to HDL-C ratios than men. At puberty, lipid levels do not change in females, but males show a significant drop in their HDL-C levels, resulting in a gender difference in this risk-lowering lipid that is maintained throughout the reproductive years. LDL-C levels change little in men but rise with age in women, so that LDL-C levels in females exceed levels in males after the age of 50, which is approximately the age of menopause. Prospective studies of women before and after the menopause have indicated that HDL-C levels decline while total cholesterol (and presumably LDL-C) levels rise by 5 percent during menopause, implicating changes in levels of reproductive hormones as important influences. These findings suggest that the increase in coronary mortality which occurs in women after the age of 65 may be due in part to the decrease in HDL-C levels as a consequence of age and menopause.

Public health initiatives to lower plasma cholesterol levels through changes in diet and, in individuals with substantial elevations, through anticholesterolemic drugs have been promoted primarily in the US. Cholesterol reduction efforts have been shown to reduce coronary mortality in men, although total mortality is not reduced (Muldoon *et al.*, 1990). For the same reasons as mentioned with regard to blood pressure, definitive evidence of the postulated benefits of such reductions in cholesterol in women are not yet available. Additional investigations which in-corporate proportionately more women than men as participants and which focus on the elderly age group are needed to clarify whether cholesterol reduction does decrease either coronary death or overall mortality among women.

Diabetes Mellitus

As a risk factor for coronary heart disease, diabetes mellitus is unusual in that this disorder conveys a higher risk for women than for men (Eaker *et al.*, 1987). This may be due in part to the observation that HDL-C levels are reduced in diabetic patients, particularly diabetic women, so that diabetes may blunt the female advantage conveyed by this risk-reducing lipid factor.

The Beaver County Study, which is the only study to date to include diabetic women and men, did not find insulin levels to be predictors of morbidity (Eaker *et al.*, 1987). In this same study, a higher insulin level was related to higher diastolic blood pressure and lower HDL-C levels in men but not women. This apparent difference may reflect a true gender difference in relationships. Alternatively, it may simply reflect the added variability induced by phase of the menstrual cycle in women where data collections occurred at different points in this cycle.

BEHAVIORAL FACTORS INFLUENCING CORONARY HEALTH AND DISEASE OUTCOMES IN WOMEN

Cigarette Smoking

For decades, cigarette smoking was more common in men than women. This gender difference has recently diminished in the US, in part because men are quitting cigarette smoking at a higher rate than women and because in the younger age groups, the proportion of women who smoke has actually increased (Gritz, 1991). This situation is creating serious concern, because cigarette smoking is a major risk factor for heart disease in both women and men and because this added risk can be avoided. Furthermore, smoking appears to compound the effect of other risk factors (high cholesterol, diabetes, hypertension, obesity), which are less easily modified. Also, unlike interventions to reduce hypertension and high cholesterol, investigations comparing cardiovascular outcomes in persons who do versus do not smoke have confirmed that quitting smoking or never smoking are associated with lower coronary death and lower total mortality in women as well as men (Eaker *et al.*, 1987; Rosenberg, 1987).

Cigarette smoking is complexly related to reproductive hormones in women. Smoking decreases natural production of estrogens and increases the rate of metabolism of those estrogens produced, leaving less available for normal functions. On average, women who smoke reach menopause at a younger age than women who never smoke. Cigarette smoking also appears to decrease the effectiveness of estrogens administered as replacement for natural estrogens after menopause or as oral contraceptives (Willett *et al.*, 1983). The combination of cigarette smoking and oral contraceptive use is a particularly negative pairing. Early studies of oral contraceptive use suggested this use led to an increased risk of myocardial infarction. Later, when newer oral contraceptive drugs with lower estradiol and progesterone dosages replaced earlier drugs, the relationship was re-examined. The results indicate that oral contraceptives by themselves do not increase risk, but that smokers who use oral contraceptives face a risk of a heart attack up to 40 times greater than other women of the same age (Rosenberg *et al.*, 1985; Stampfer *et al.*, 1990). This enhanced risk appears to involve the synthetic ethinylestradiol component of these drugs which increase lever production of factors promoting coagulation and thus thrombo-embolism; natural estrogens used in postmenopausal replacement therapy do not have this adverse effect.

The message about the health risks of cigarette smoking is widely known So, why do women in particular continue to smoke? One major factor appears to be the social emphasis placed on being thin and lean for women today. Smokers weigh less than nonsmokers on average and quitting frequently leads to weight gain. This fact may encourage young women wanting to be more attractive to begin smoking and it certainly sabotages efforts to quit for many women. Women who smoke also exercise less than nonsmokers, which tends to decrease their ability to control weight and slimness by that means (Gritz *et al.*, 1989; Gritz, 1991). Another factor may be the stress reduction aspect to smoking. Many women who combine full-time work outside the home with the unpaid hours spent working as a housewife and mother have little time left for themselves to seek recreation or stress reducing activities. Cigarette smoking induces a sense of relaxation both because of the physiological effects of the nicotine and deep inhalation and because of learned association with moments of relaxation (coffee breaks etc.), yet it takes only a few minutes or can even be done while driving, cooking or performing many other routine activities. To promote smoking cessation or never smoking, new messages and new learning must replace these old patterns: 1) smoking is unattractive, no matter how much thinner you are; and 2) other relaxation techniques can be learned and practiced effectively in the few minutes required for smoking. These challenges must be addressed to reduce the excess risk of heart disease in women which continues to result from cigarette smoking.

Obesity and Exercise Patterns

Obesity is a risk factor for heart disease in both women and men and its effects may be particularly enhanced in combination with other risk factors, particularly hypertension and diabetes. Even so, recently health practitioners have begun to question whether women as a group should be encouraged to initiate weight reduction efforts. In part, this concern is based on the relatively low success rate achieved by most weight loss interventions. Of those women who achieve a reduction of 20 pounds or more in such interventions, 60–70 percent will fail to maintain their loss over a two-year period. There is concern that repeated cycles of weight loss and gain may enhance certain health risks while achieving no sustained weight reduction in most individuals (Jeffery, 1991). There is also concern that failure to maintain weight losses may lead to maladaptive outcomes, such as cigarette smoking or depression, which are likely to be associated with increased rather than decreased morbidity and mortality. Further study of the health impact of weight fluctuation is needed. Nevertheless, it is clear that efforts aimed at weight reduction in women are unlikely to yield clearly positive effects on cardiovascular health except in the minority of participants who achieve and maintain weight losses without altering other risk factors.

In contrast to the limited success predicted for weight loss interventions, efforts to increase physical activity have a substantial record of success. Increasing physical activity reduces risk of coronary heart disease mortality in men and women. In addition, enhanced activity is effective in smokers as well as nonsmokers; a smoker who is very active and fit appears to have approximately the same risk of heart disease as a nonsmoker who is totally sedentary. Furthermore, recent observations indicate that although very active and fit people are at lowest risk, the greatest difference in risk of coronary mortality is seen when comparing totally sedentary people to moderately active people. Thus, great risk reduction can be achieved by only a modest increase in activity in people who have been very inactive. Also, one recent study indicated that frequent short bouts of exercise (20–30 minutes several times per week) and less frequent long bouts of exercise (>40 minutes, 1–2 times per week) had equal benefits in reducing risk (King, 1991).

Still, data indicate that 75 percent of women in the US are irregularly active or totally sedentary. This large percentage indicates that, for women, there are a number of social barriers to overcome in efforts to increase physical activity. Finding time to exercise is a challenge for many women who have both a full-time job and a home and family to maintain. Since creating this time may require some accommodation by the male members of the household, it is important that men be informed both about the link between physical activity and reduced risk of heart disease and the fact that this disorder is the major killer of women as well as men. Also, home-based aerobic exercise programs which can be accomplished through television, videotapes or moderately priced equipment such as exercise bicycles, step platforms, skiing and rowing machines and so on, may prove to be the best choices for women whose free time does not fall in daylight hours or who cannot easily travel to a health club.

Behavioral Patterns: Type A, Hostility, Depression and Lack of Social Support

It has long been hypothesized that certain personality traits or behavioral patterns may predispose the individual to develop coronary disease. The most widely discussed example of this is the Type A behavior pattern, exemplified by a person high in hostility, competitiveness and time urgency. Prospective longitudinal research has been inconsistent in regard to relationships between Type A and coronary morbidity and mortality. However, cross-sectional studies with large samples including women as well as men have documented that Type A is associated with early development of coronary artery occlusion in both women and men, but not with coronary disease in older participants (Williams *et al.*, 1988). Similarly, hostility (whether measured with Type A in the Structured Interview or independently by questionnaire) has been found to be associated with coronary occlusion in young women and men, particularly those under the age of 50 (Barefoot *et al.*, 1991). In the prospec-tive Western Electric Study, high hostility predicted increased coronary deaths and total mortality. Hostility has also been associated with higher LDL-C and total cholesterol in men and women (Weidner *et al.*, 1987). It is important to note that Type A may primarily be associated with coronary disease because of its hostility component. Also, both Type A and hostility are associated with greater cigarette smoking and alcohol con-sumption, so that care must be taken to adjust for these differences when assessing the link between personality patterns and heart disease.

Depression is another behavioral trait which has been associated with coronary heart disease, including sudden cardiac death and myocardial infarction (eg. Carney *et al.*, 1989). Although most of these data were obtained cross-sectionally or retrospectively and women were not included as participants in many of the studies, depression is nevertheless hypothesized to relate strongly to heart disease in women. This is because the prevalence of clinical depression is substantially higher in women compared to men. In addition, while major depression typically is found in 20 percent of male patients with a history of myocardial infarction or documented coronary disease, it has been observed in 50 percent of females having a history of infarction and 30 percent of females with coronary disease. Finally, one study from Iowa which followed nearly 3,000 women psychiatric patients for over 4 years compared to other patient groups found that deaths from heart disease were increased in these patients, most of whom had depression; a similar comparison involving male psychiatric and non-psychiatric patients did not show an enhanced risk of coronary mortality (Carney, 1991).

Although the evidence does suggest that Type A, hostility and depression may all predispose women to develop greater coronary heart disease, prospective studies which follow women with and without these behavioral traits who are initially disease-free over periods of many years are needed to confirm these relationships. In addition, considerable research should be initiated to determine whether interventions designed to alter these behavioral patterns are effective in reducing risk of coronary mortality in women. Interventions combining relaxation training and education about Type A behaviors in group settings have been found to reduce re-infarction rates in Type A men who have had a previous myocardial infarction (Friedman *et al.*, 1984). Stress management training is also currently being used with men and women having documented coronary disease who have anxiety and depression, with the aim of reducing risk of future infarctions. More of such intervention projects focusing on women as well as men are clearly needed.

Social support is another important behavioral influence on risk for coronary heart disease in both women and men. The basic elements of social support are having a network of friends, family, co-workers and so on who provide a variety of social resources, including affection, listening/communiction, material aid, and feelings of belonging. Social support is generally viewed as an exchange process, with each person who is involved functioning as both a recipient and a provider of support, although one of these roles may tend to dominate in any given social relationship.

A number of major prospective studies have linked lack of good social support to coronary mortality as well as mortality from all causes; these studies have been summarized in recent comprehensive review articles by Shumaker and Hill (1991) and by Berkman (1991). In the Alameda County, California investigation, both being unmarried or widowed and having few contacts with friends and relatives increased risk of death in men and women from the age of 30 upward, but lack of marital support was more strongly related for men while lack of support from family and friends was more strongly related for women. In the Tecumseh (Michigan) Community Health Study, lesser overall social support was related to death from coronary heart disease but not all cause mortality in women, although this social index was related to both outcomes in men. In this investigation and in the Evans County, Georgia study, which yielded a relationship to overall mortality in white men and women, the primary effect was due to differences between participants who had essentially no social contacts versus those who had some social network. Subjects with moderate versus high social support did not differ. Similar findings have been obtained in recent investigations in Sweden and Finland. Based on the Swedish National Survey of Living Conditions, both men and women in the lowest social support groups had higher coronary-related and total deaths that those in moderate or high social support groups, who did not differ from each other. In the North Karelia, Finland study, the same relationships were obtained except that the effect was weaker in women than men, yielding only a nonsignificant trend in the expected direction.

The mechanisms through which social support influences coronary health and disease are not known, but these may differ between women and men (Waldron and Jacobs, 1989). One psychophysiological hypothesis is that social support may buffer individuals from episodically high cardiovascular reactions to life stressors. Some, but not all, laboratory studies have indicated that the presence of a friend can reduce such reactions to challenging mental tasks (Kamark *et al.*, 1990; Gerin *et al.*, 1992). Possible gender differences in such effects of social support need further exploration. Another hypothesis is that social support reduces both hostility and depression and acts in part by attenuating risk associated with these characteristics. These two explanations are not mutually exclusive, but may both be true.

High Cardiovascular Reactivity to Stress

An underlying assumption of most research focusing on cardiovascular changes during behavioral events is that those individuals who show above average increases in cardiac or blood pressure measures are at greater risk of developing hypertension and coronary heart disease. This assumption, which has been labeled 'The Reactivity Hypothesis', has been supported by a few recent prospective studies. In one study of male physicians who were formerly students at Johns Hopkins Medical School, those who as students had fallen in the top 25 percent in terms of their systolic pressure increase to the painful immersion of one hand in ice and water (cold pressor test) demonstrated higher incidence of hypertension over the next 15–30 years than less reactive participants (Menkes *et al.*, 1989). Similarly, in Italy, young men and women with borderline hypertension who showed greater diastolic pressure increases during and for five minutes after a mental arithmetic task were found to develop sustained hypertension more frequently than those less reactive (Borghi *et al.*, 1986). Finally, in our own research laboratory, men who showed greater heart rate and blood pressure increases to a reaction time task as college students were found 10 years later to demonstrate higher blood pressure levels at work and at home, as well as during clinical-type stethoscopic determinations (Light *et al.*, 1992). Although positive findings from additional studies would be more convincing, this evidence is supportive of the Reactivity Hypothesis for men; however, women were involved in only one of these studies and then in too few numbers to determine whether the relationship obtained was similarly strong for both genders.

In contrast to these few prospective studies, hundreds of cross-sectional studies have compared cardiovascular responses to behavioral stressors in men and women. The results have confirmed quite consistently that men demonstrate greater systolic pressure increases than women to a variety of stressors (Stoney *et al.*, 1987). Studies in children and adolescents have confirmed that this gender difference in systolic reactivity is absent in children age 7–14, but evident in those 15 years and older, who are usually past puberty. Diastolic pressure and heart rate responses are not greater in males and many studies have reported greater heart rate increases in females (Matthews and Stoney, 1988). In recent studies, noninvasive assessment of cardiac output or the amount of blood pumped by the heart each minute has been possible. One study comparing women in nontraditional career training (medicine, dentistry, law, science) with men observed greater cardiac output increases to stress among the women (Girdler *et al.*, 1990). Another study using a broader sample of white collar and blue collar male and female workers indicated no consistent gender differences in cardiac output response (Light *et al.*, in press). These findings are of interest because cardiac output is both a determinant of blood pressure and an indication of how hard the heart is working during stressors.

The physiological mechanisms behind these gender differences in cardiovascular reactivity to stressors may involve the adrenal hormones, adrenaline and noradrenaline (epinephrine and norepinephrine), and/or the sympathetic (adrenergic) receptors on the heart and in the blood vessels. Swedish women have been shown to exhibit lesser increases in levels of adrenaline during important examinations and at work than their male counterparts (Frankenhaeuser, 1983). In a study by Freedman, Sabharwal and Desai (1987), men were shown to demonstrate greater vascular constriction and dilation than women in response to specific drugs which stimulate the alpha and beta adrenergic receptors in those blood vessels. These observations suggest that women may show lesser blood pressure increases to stress than men because their adrenergic receptors in blood vessels are less sensitive or less dense. Further study comparing receptor sensitivity in men and women and relating any differences in such sensitivity to observations of blood pressure reactivity to stress in the same individuals is needed to confirm this suggestion. Also, the long-term significance of these differences, particularly whether receptor sensitivity and reactivity differences contribute to the relatively protected status of women in relation to coronary disease, needs to be established.

REPRODUCTIVE HORMONES AS POSSIBLE MECHANISMS INFLUENCING CARDIOVASCULAR HEALTH AND DISEASE IN WOMEN

Menopause and Estrogen Replacement Therapy

The sharp rise in the rate of development of coronary disease in women after age 50–55 led many authorities to focus on the menopause and the hormonal transition which occurs at that time as sources of this change in coronary risk. Two-thirds of women pass through the menopause between the ages of 48 and 53; during this interval of only 5 years, coronary mortality rates in females increase by over 100 percent (Stampfer *et al.*, 1990). Nonetheless, this is an association with age, not menopause per se. Additional research comparing women before and after menopause is essential to draw direct conclusions. Furthermore, such studies must appropriately adjust for age, obesity and smoking, which are known to influence both coronary risk and menopausal status.

The Framingham Heart Study examined the effects of natural menopause in nearly 2,000 women who were examined every 2 years for a period of up to 26 years (Lerner and Kannel, 1986). Although the relative risk of coronary heart disease was roughly twice as great in post-menopausal versus pre-menopausal women, since there were only 18 cases of this disease altogether even over the long follow-up time, the finding appears statistically unstable. In a much larger prospective investigation involving over 116,000 female nurses (Colditz *et al.*, 1987), the Nurses Health Study indicated that fatal and nonfatal coronary disease occurred nearly three times as often in naturally postmenopausal women as compared to premenopausal women matched for age within a 5-year range. When matched within a 1-year age range and matched for smoking habits as well, however, this difference disappeared. In contrast to natural menopause, surgical removal of the ovaries in this same study was associated with a doubling of coronary risk even after precise adjustment for age and smoking. These results were interpreted as indicating that the ovaries and ovarian hormones are important contributers to the relatively protected status of women against coronary disease and fatality. However, in natural menopause, the decrease in ovarian function occurs gradually, a decline beginning before and continuing after termination of menses. Thus, the occurrence of menopause does not evoke an abrupt change in risk for coronary disease, although with the gradual decline in ovarian function beginning before menopause, a period of increasing risk has begun. It may take many years for the consequences of this change to be reflected in changes in coronary health outcomes (Stampfer *et al.*, 1990).

The greatest support for this interpretation of the importance of menopause derives in fact from studies of the effects of providing estrogen supplements to replace natural estrogens after menopause. Stampfer and Colditz (1991) recently reviewed numerous published cross-sectional and prospective investigations, including the Lipid Research Clinic Follow-up, the Framingham Heart Study and the Nurses Health Study. Their conclusion is that estrogen replacement therapy cuts risks of coronary death in half, independent of age or other risk factors. They do report that adjusting for HDL-C and LDL-C levels results in a weaker effect; however, such an adjustment is probably not appropriate in any case since estrogen's primary mechanism of action may be through alterations in specific cholesterol concentrations.

In his recent review, Lobo (1990) cites evidence that estrogen replacement therapy lowers LDL-C and total cholesterol, while increasing the beneficial HDL-C levels. Also, evidence is presented suggesting that estrogen may directly affect vessel walls, increasing the vasodilation and blood flow. Interestingly, progestins appear to act in an opposing manner, tending to lower HDL-C levels and to inhibit estrogen's positive effects on blood vessels. Lobo argues quite convincingly that, because so many more female lives are lost due to heart disease than to other causes, like breast or endometrial cancer, estrogen should be prescribed widely for postmenopausal women even though there may be slight increases in risk of these latter disorders associated with use of estrogen without progestin. According to his figures, 328 lives will be saved from coronary deaths per 100,000 women if estrogen supplements are used as compared with only 65 lives saved from cancer if estrogen supplements are not used. Progestins, which appear to protect against estrogen's increase in risk of endometrial cancer only, were not recommended for use together with estrogen since they are expected to reduce the lives saved from coronary disease by 117 lives compared to only 27 lives saved by preventing endometrial cancer.

Ovarian Hormones, Behavioral Patterns and Cardiovascular Responses to Stress

In her recent position paper, Matthews (1989) contends that when considered separately, neither the biological nor the behavioral risk factors as currently assessed can fully account for the observed gender difference in risk of coronary heart disease. After statistical adjustment for blood pressure, plasma glucose, obesity, cholesterol, smoking, marital status, education and age, the Rancho Bernardo study (Wingard *et al.*, 1983) showed that the relative risk in men versus women fell from 4.8 times to 2.4 times but did not become equal. How, then, can we explain the cardiovascular benefit of being female? Matthews proposes that rather than being a simple sum of the lower risk factors mentioned above which are associated with being a woman, the benefits derive from this sum plus the interaction between biological and behavioral factors.

Female gender, thus, may lower risk in three ways: 1) by lessening exposure to adverse environmental factors; 2) by modifying the individual's psycho-physiological responses to such exposure; and 3) by modifying the relationship of any specific risk factor to disease development by modifying the balance of all risk factors entering the predictive equation.

A limited quantity of research by Matthews and by other scientists has evaluated psychophysiological responses in interaction with female ovarian hormones. A number of these studies have compared cardiovascular and hormonal responses to standard physical and mental tasks in young women during different phases of their menstrual cycles. Most studies comparing phase effects within the same women have found no differences in the magnitude of blood presure or heart rate increases between the early follicular phase of the cycle (when estrogen and progesterone are low) versus the late luteal phase (when estrogen and progesterone are high). In our most recent effort, we observed this similarity of blood pressure reactivity, but found that there were still important cardiovascular differences (Girdler *et al.*, 1992). In the luteal (higher hormone) phase, women showed greater increases in the heart's stroke volume (blood pumped per beat) but lesser vascular resistance (construction of vessels) during stress, than the same women showed during the follicular (low hormone) phase. These cardiovascular patterns suggest that the changes in estrogen/progesterone balance in women over the normal monthly cycle may complexly modulate responses of the heart and blood vessels to arousal induced by stress exposure.

Other research has compared cardiovascular stress responses in pre-versus post-menopausal women. Postmenopausal women were found to show consistently greater heart rate increases and greater systolic pressure and adrenaline increases during a simulated public speech compared to premenopausal women. It is not clear at present whether such enhanced cardiovascular reactivity after menopause is a reproducible finding, or whether this effect might be minimized by use of estrogen replacement therapy. Resting blood pressure has also been shown to be lower or unchanged in most women using estrogen replacement therapy roughly 5 percent may show blood pressure increases (Lobo, 1990). Studies of younger women taking estrogens and progestins in the form of oral contraceptives have indicated that this form of hormonal therapy may enhance blood pressure responses to stress but only among cigarette smokers and women with a family history of heart disease. It is also important to emphasize that the synthetic estrogens used in formulating oral contraceptives are different from the natural estrogens (conjugated equine estrogen, estradiol, estrone) in their effects on coagulation, and may differ in other cardiovascular effects as well.

Some of the most intriguing observations indicating interactions between gender, behavior and coronary heart disease have been obtained in monkeys. Among male cynomolgus monkeys fed a high fat diet, those who are socially dominant yet forced to live in unstable social groups by frequently moving them to new groups demonstrated greater coronary artery disease than other males (Kaplan *et al.*, 1982). Normal females who are dominant show much less occlusion of coronary vessels under these same unstable conditions, but if these dominant females have had their ovaries removed, they too demonstrate a dramatic increase in coronary disease (Adams *et al.*, 1985). Most interesting are the subordinate or low social status female monkeys. Even in a stable social setting, these females are stressed by spending more time in isolation and submitting to aggressive behavior by others. This increased stress (confirmed by evidence of chronic cortisol elevations) has been interpreted as the source of poor ovarian function in subordinate females; they have lower estrogen and progestin levels and more frequently have anovulatory cycles compared to dominant females. Exactly how stress exposure may act to decrease levels of ovarian hormones is not yet known. What is known is that these subordinate female monkeys demonstrate increased coronary artery occlusion, which can be prevented by administering estrogen supplements. Although parallels between human and monkey social behavior are certainly imperfect, it is noteworthy that among males the aggressive, hostile, dominant subgroup develops greater coronary disease, while among females the socially isolated, behaviorally depressed subgroup is more vulnerable to coronary disease. Future research in humans may clarify whether behavioral patterns involving chronic exposure to stress, hostility, isolation and depression also lead to different health outcomes in men and women.

SUMMARY

There are many positive themes in the current literature on women and cardiovascular health and disease. Naturally, the confirmation of the lower risk of coronary disease in women, especially young women, is welcome. Knowledge about how various risk factors relate specifically to women of various ages has grown, and further progress is expected soon. Even more positive are the recent insights into the beneficial effects of natural ovarian hormones and hormone replacement in improving cholesterol levels, and lowering risk of coronary disease and death. This information may be useful in saving the lives of women in this present decade. Foundations are in place for further study of the menopause and of behavioral patterns which may relate to differential coronary health outcomes. Plans for further interventions in addition to estrogen therapy and smoking cessation programs may be designed focusing on increasing physical activity and decreasing physiological reactions to life stressors.

As another important sign of progress, we also wish to emphasize the growing awareness among medical practitioners that the study of women's health and disease processes requires special attention. We cannot assume that the patterns and relationships obtained by studying men will be fully descriptive for women as well; such an approach would totally ignore ovarian hormones, which now are a well-documented factor in coronary health of women. Dr. Bernadine Healy of the U.S. National Institutes of Health cited two recent studies indicating gender bias in medical treatment, showing that women received less angiography, angioplasty or by-pass surgery than men when they were admitted to hospital with coronary symptoms. However, when a woman had a documented myocardial infarction, her treatment would be just like a man's. Dr. Healy called this treatment bias "the Yentl Syndrome", after a Jewish story heroine who must pretend to be a man to be allowed to become a scholar. We concur with Healy (1991) when she makes this compelling challenge to all physicians and scientists: "We must be challenged by the example of coronary artery disease to examine critically the extent to which the Yentl syndrome pervades medicine and medical research... Indeed, it is now time for a general awakening. Women have unique medical problems... Although women live longer than men – by as much as seven years on average – the quality of life of those extra years is exceptionally burdened by cancer, particularly of the breast, lung and colon, by heart disease and stroke, osteoporosis, Alzheimer's disease, depression and social isolation, and general frailty. These conditions . . . are not the inevitable ravages of age but are in many cases highly preventable and eminently treatable. We must awaken fully to these facts and address the diseases of women as different from the diseases of men but of equal importance, even when they also affect men" (p. 275).

FURTHER READING

Amastos, K., Charney, P., Charon, R.A., Cohen, E., Jones, C.Y., Marte, C., Swiderski, D.M., Wheat, M.E. and Williams, S. (1991). Hypertension in women: What is really known? Report of The Women's Caucus, Working Group on Women's Health of the Society of General Internal Medicine. *Annals of Internal Medicine*, 115, 287–293.

Eaker, E.A., Packard, B., Wenger, N.K., Clarkson, T.B. and Tyroler, H.A. (1987). Coronary heart disease in women: Reviewing the evidence, identifying the needs: A summary of the proceedings. Administrative report. Bethesda, MD: National Heart, Lung, and Blood Institute, National Institutes of Health, pp. 1–48.

Healy, B. (1991). The Yentl Syndrome. *New England Journal of Medicine*, 325, 274–276.

Lobo, R.A. (1990). Estrogen and cardiovascular disease. *Annals of the New York Academy of Sciences*, 592, 286–294.

6

CANCER

BARBARA L. ANDERSEN

Department of Psychology, Ohio State University, 1885 Neil Avenue, Columbus, Ohio 43210-1222, USA

Each year approximately one million Americans develop cancer and half a million die of the disease (Boring *et al.*, 1992). Countries differ in their prevalence and death rates for cancer. For example, England and Wales have the fourth highest death rate in the world for women with cancer, with 164 women per 100,000 dying each year. However disturbing these figures are, they can be contrasted with other data, such as a 1989 *Lancet* report of the long term (10 year) follow-up of women with recurrent breast cancer who participated in a group therapy intervention. David Spiegel, Joan Bloom and their colleagues (Spiegel, *et al.*, 1989) reported mortality data for 50 intervention and 36 no treatment control women. The women in the intervention group had participated in a group support intervention to enhance adjustment and reduce disease symptoms, such as pain. Their earlier research found that the intervention had helped the women feel less depressed, fatigued and troubled by the chronic pain from their illness. These and related reports had suggested that gains could be achieved with psychological therapy, even as life ebbs away. However, the dramatic data in the follow up showed an 18 month survival time difference between the groups, a mean of 36.6 months for the intervention and 18.9 months for the control, indicating that the women receiving the psychological intervention lived significantly longer. Findings such as these have renewed interest in a role for psychological efforts in coping and living with cancer.

This chapter provides a brief overview of the cancer problem for women and summarizes the psychological and behavioral aspects. We will first describe the major disease sites for women. The psychological data will then be grouped into disease-relevant time points, from diagnosis to recovery and death, but we will begin with prevention efforts with women.

COMMON MALIGNANCIES: INCIDENCE, RISK FACTORS, TREATMENT, AND SURVIVAL

Among adult females cancer is a leading cause of death, usually ranking either first or second across age groups. The top cancer killers of women; lung, colo-rectal, breast and gynecologic cancer, account for approximately 70 percent of all cancers in women. Cancers vary in the prevalence and mortality. Table 6.1 displays data from the US on the incidence and death rates for specific sites. These data indicate, for example, that the breast is the most common site for disease, but lung cancer kills the most women.

TABLE 6.1

Cancer Incidence and Deaths in Women by Site – 1992 Estimates

Incidence (Total est. 565,000)			Deaths (Total est. 245,000)		
Site	Number	Percentage	Site	Number	Percentage
Breast	180,000	32%	Lung	53,000	21%
Colon/Rectum	77,000	17%	Breast	46,000	18%
Lung	66,000	12%	Colon/Rectum	29,400	12%
Uterus	45,500	8%	Pancreas	13,000	5%
Lymphoma	21,200	4%	Ovary	13,000	5%
Ovary	21,000	4%	Uterus	10,000	4%
Melanoma	15,000	3%	Lymphoma	10,000	4%
Pancreas	14,400	3%	Leukemia	8,300	3%
Bladder	13,100	2%	Liver	5,700	2%
Leukemia	12,200	2%	Brain	5,300	2%
Kidney	10,300	2%	Stomach	5,300	2%
Oral	9,700	2%	Mul. Myeloma	4,500	2%

Adapted from Cancer Facts & Figures – 1992. (1992). American Cancer Society, Inc.

TABLE 6.2

Age-Adjusted Death Rates in Females Per 100,000 Population
for Selected Sites for Selected Countries

Country	All Sites	Lung	Breast	Colon/Rectum	Uterus
United States	109.7 (7)	22.7	22.4	12.0	2.7
Canada	111.5 (5)	19.5	24.2	12.9	2.5
Denmark	139.4 (1)	22.3	28.3	17.5	3.6
England & Wales	126.9 (2)	20.1	29.3	14.2	2.6
France	89.9 (12)	4.8	19.6	10.6	4.3
Germany (Dem)	102.9 (8)	5.7	17.2	14.5	4.0
Ireland	126.1 (3)	17.7	27.0	16.6	2.9
Italy	99.7 (9)	7.2	20.6	10.3	2.8
Netherlands	110.0 (6)	9.1	26.8	13.7	2.6
North Ireland	123.0 (4)	17.5	27.0	16.5	2.6
Sweden	98.6 (10)	9.5	17.4	11.2	2.6
USSR	92.9 (11)	6.9	12.9	10.6	4.3

Note: Figures in parentheses are order of rank within site.
Adapted from Cancer Facts & Figures – 1992. (1992). American Cancer Society, Inc.

Similarly, Table 6.2 provides death rate data from selected Western countries, which indicates that there are considerable geographic and nationality differences. Examine the differences, for example, between England/Wales and the Netherlands in the death rates due to lung cancer (rates of 20 vs 9 per 100,000 women, respectively).

Breast

Several variables have been identified as risk factors for breast cancer. The demographics of age (age increases risk), race (white women have higher risk), ethnicity (Jewish women have higher rates), and income (the highest socioeconomic status groups have greater risk) have been studied. Family history is critical, as women who are daughters or siblings of women with breast cancer are at almost three times the risk. Study of reproductive history indicates that women who have no pregnancy or have their first child after the age of 30 have almost a threefold increase in risk as compared to those giving birth the first time at age 20 or younger. Breast cancer is usually first discovered as a painless, mobile lump by the woman or her physician. It usually spreads locally, by moving directly into the surrounding breast tissue and eventually involving the overlying skin or the underlying muscle. As many as 40–50 percent of patients have progressed and have disease in the nearby lymph nodes at diagnosis.

A century ago in 1894 the primary treatment for breast cancer, radical mastectomy, was described by Halsted and Meyer. The procedure consisted of removal of the entire breast as well as the underlying and surrounding muscles, leaving a significant chest wall defect. By 1970, controversy surrounding surgical management was apparent and randomized clinical trials were begun. Results indicated that there were no differences between groups in survival times – indicating that less radical surgery (ie. modified radical mastectomy with or without radiotherapy) could significantly reduce unpleasant side effects (eg. problems with arm mobility, body image) without compromising mortality. Also, breast reconstruction was possible with less dramatic (ie. radical) surgery. Since breast cancer often spreads to the surrounding areas at diagnosis, additional therapy – usually chemotherapy or hormonal therapy is often included.

Colon and Rectum

Incidence rates of colorectal cancer among men and women and among white and black females are comparable (Bean, 1986). Risk factors include age, personal or family history of cancer, or history of bowel diseases such as polyps or inflammatory bowel disease. Currently, early detection strategies include stool blood slide tests, rectal examination and proctosigmoidoscopy. Symptoms are often vague and insidious; they may only come late in the disease and are primarily related to the location of the tumor. Right sided lesions tend to be bulky but they do not cause early symptoms and chronic bleeding may go unnoticed. In contrast, left sided lesions may produce change in bowel habits (eg. constipation) with visible blood in the stool. Rectal lesions may produce pain and discomfort.

Bowel tumors penetrate progressively through the bowel wall, spread regionally by the lymphatic system and, with distant spread, cells are shed into the gastrointestinal tract. Nearly 80 percent of patients will be candidates for surgery, with or without radiation therapy.

Lung

There has been a striking increase in incidence of lung cancer among women. Smoking is considered to be the major etiologic agent as the increase is directly related to women's changed smoking patterns in the 1940's, 50's, and 60's. For example, Higgins (1984) in the US reported that in 1935 only 18 percent of the female population smoked, but in 1955 the prevalence was 25 percent and it climbed to 33 percent in 1965 (Bean, 1986). Since 1987 in the US, more women have annually died of lung than breast cancer, a trend which is expected to continue for at least the next 15–20 years.

Clinical presentation of lung cancer varies and mimics other pulmonary conditions. Symptoms/signs include cough, wheezing and pain on breathing. Lung cancer can also produce symptoms remote from the disease. Untreated, 95 percent of lung cancer patients will die within 1 year. Even with treatment, the 5-year survival rate (ie. the number of diagnosed patients who are still alive 5 years following treatment) is approximately 12 percent (Boring, et al., 1992). Aggressive surgery is the treatment of choice for all patients except those with small cell carcinomas which are treated with chemotherapy. For those with advanced disease, treatment has included a variety of chemotherapy regimens and a patient must consider the costs and benefits of the side effects of the chemotherapies relative to the expected duration and quality of her life.

Gynecologic Cancer

There are four major sites for gynecologic cancer: the endometrium (accounting for 46 percent of all the new cases), ovary (29 percent), cervix (18 percent), and the vulva (5 percent, which also includes the remaining others, such as the fallopian tube).

Endometrium

The most frequent complaint that brings a woman to medical attention is post-menopausal vaginal bleeding or perimenopausal abnormal bleeding; pelvic pain is occasionally reported. Endometrial cancer rates show a sharp increase in the perimenopausal years, with a peak occurrence between the ages of 55 and 66. A variety of data suggests that estrogenic stimulation is linked to etiology. According to this viewpoint, stimulation could be increased and/or decreased through endogenous sources (eg. peripheral estrone which is high among post menopausal and/or obese women) and exogenous sources (eg. estrogen replacement therapy following meno-pause). Treatment for endometrial cancer usually consists of total abdominal hysterectomy and bilateral salpingo-oophorectomy (TAH-BSO) ie. removal of uterus, ovaries and fallopian tubes, radiation therapy, or a combination with hormone therapy.

Ovary

This is the most frustrating and discouraging of gynecologic diseases for physicians. The causes of the disease are not clear. Ovary disease accounts for only 4 percent of all cancers in women, but it has the fourth highest death rate and the rate has remained stable despite numbers of clinical studies with chemotherapy agents. Patients typically come to their physician with vague, nonspecific symptoms of short duration (eg. abdominal swelling, pain, nausea, or vaginal bleeding). Only one-fourth are diagnosed with limited disease, compared to 50 to 80 percent of women with other types of gynecologic cancer. Treatment usually consists of TAH-BSO followed by lengthy and toxic chemotherapy regimens.

Cervix

Once the most common gynecologic malignancy, cervix cancer has had a world-wide decline in incidence, perhaps due to the increased usage of Pap smear screening. Extensive epidemiologic data exist, with the search for a sexually transmissible agent as a major focus. Early age at first intercourse and the number of different sexual partners at an early age may be influential along with intercourse with 'high risk' males (ie. a male who has had contact with multiple partners). Treatment strategies for cervical cancer are similar to those for endometrial disease. For those with recurrent disease or extensive disease at diagnosis, the scenario is much more difficult and may include radical pelvic surgery.

Vulva

This cancer is a rare one and occurs most commonly among older women, with a median age of 65 years for white and 55 years for black women. When a woman seeks treatment, vulvar itching is often a longstanding complaint, although a mass or growth is most common. Ignorance or misinterpretation of the symptoms is common for patients and physicans alike such that delay is a major problem. Treatment is often a modified radical vulvectomy, which removes labial tissue and often the clitoris and usually the lymph nodes in the groins and/or pelvis. Radiation therapy has played a limited role in treatment. This treatment can produce extreme genital disfigurement and many women have difficulty adjusting to the body changes (Anderson and Hacker, 1983).

PSYCHOLOGICAL AND BEHAVIORAL ASPECTS: FROM DIAGNOSIS THROUGH RECOVERY OR DEATH

Prevention

It has been suggested that much of cancer incidence and premature death can be prevented through changes in behavior. In the United States, for example, the National Cancer Institute (NCI) has set a goal of a 50 percent reduction in cancer mortality by the year 2000 through prevention and control efforts focussed, to a large extent, on life style (Greenwald and Cullen, 1985).

Primary prevention attempts to reduce the probability of cancer onset by decreasing exposure to risk factors. For women and men, unhealthy habits have been a behavioral research target and smoking has been emphasized as it is believed to be related to 30 percent of all cancer deaths. (Cigarette smoking is directly linked to lung cancer, the leading cause of death for men and women, and is implicated in cancers of the larynx, head and neck, esophagus, bladder, kidney, pancreas, and stomach). The other major categories of lifestyle behavior that have been linked to greater risk are diet (including alcohol usage) and sun exposure. In the area of diet, the majority of the research has dealt with diet modification and weight reduction, per se. In contrast, there has been less behavioral research on the hazards of solar exposure, despite the importance of epidemiologic studies which provided prevention information (eg. the most damaging ultraviolet exposure occurs during the midday sun).

Psychologists have contributed to *secondary prevention* efforts, identifying the disease at the earliest of stages (eg. when it is preinvasive or localized and usually asymptomatic) so that a diagnosis can be made and treatment can be administered sooner. For women, the early detection of breast cancer has been a major focus. Of the three approaches [mammography, clinical breast examination, and breast self-examination (BSE)], BSE has received the greatest behavioral study. Research has found that many women decline to participate in screening programs and variables difficult to change through intervention (eg. age, lower socioeconomic status, less familiarity with the health care system, and less-positive attitudes toward medical care) are predictive of this and related health behaviors (eg. delay to seek treatment), but there have also been small scale interventions to increase BSE performance (see Mayer and Solomon, in press, for a review). Unfortunately, data have not linked BSE to reduced cancer mortality rates. Because of this, the medical community currently regards mammography as the most reliable means of early detection, which has resulted in the expansion of behavioral research (see Rimer, 1992, for a review).

Efforts have recently begun in the area of *teritiary prevention*, shortening delay to seek a diagnosis once symptom/sign awareness has occurred. Unlike many medical problems, the development of malignancy and the appearance of symptoms are protracted and a complex and changing symptom picture can be typical. Recent studies indicate that the lion's share of delay (ie. from the symptom/sign awareness to appearing before a physician for consultation) is accounted for by the time necessary for the patient to decide that the symptoms indicate 'illness' rather than a normal and/or non serious health condition (eg. a 45-year old woman eventually decides that her irregular vaginal bleeding may indicate a serious condition such as cancer rather than a normal process such as menopause). Interestingly, the delayed 'serious' judgment also appears in the few studies of physicians' delay in making cancer diagnoses for their patients. Such data directly counter popular notions that individuals deny cancer symptomatology and/or delay due to fears of the disease or treatment.

Diagnosis

The concept of 'existential plight' has been offered to describe individual's immediate reaction and subsequent emotional turmoil (Weisman and Worden, 1976). The emotions that have been well studied are sadness (depression), fear (anxiety), and anger. Of these, depression is, not surprisingly, the most common affective problem. In an early report of hospitalized cancer patients referred for psychiatric consultation, Levin, Silberfarb, and Lipowski (1978) noted that the majority (56 percent) were depression diagnoses. More recent surveys have also cited depression as the most prevalent affective problem, but estimates of major depression are in the order of 5–6 percent (Derogatis *et al.*, 1983; Lansky *et al.*, 1985). When less severe depression and depressed mood are considered, prevalence rates are higher (eg. 16 percent in Derogatis *et al.*, 1983) but still not of the magnitude of the previous decade. In general, depression is more common for those patients in active treatment rather than those on follow-up, receiving palliative rather than curative treatment, with pain or other disturbing symptoms rather than not and with a history of affective disorder.

Several studies with female cancer patients have explored the possibility that the distress which accompanies diagnosis and the early stages of treatment can be alleviated through psychological interventions (see Andersen, in press, for a review). Two non-equivalent control group designs have provided brief interventions to gynecologic cancer patients. Capone and colleagues (1980) provided a brief, crisis-oriented intervention which assisted women to express feelings related to their diagnosis or upcoming treatments, provided information about treatment side effects and attempted to enhance self esteem, feminity and interpersonal relationships. For sexually active women, a sexual therapy component included sexual information and methods to cope and reduce anxiety when resuming intercourse. The format was at least four individual sessions during the surgical hospitalization and fifty-six newly diagnosed women participated. A non-equivalent control group was obtained by recruiting previously treated women as they returned for post-treatment follow up. Data was gathered at pre-treatment and during the first post-treatment year. Analyses indicated no differences between groups or within the intervention group on the measures of emotional distress. A trend in the percentages of women returning to work favored the intervention participants (eg. 50 percent vs. 25 percent at 3 months). In contrast to these findings, substantial differences were found between the groups in the return to and frequency of intercourse at follow up.

The second quasi-experimental investigation was reported by Houts, Whitney, Mortel and Bartholomew (1986) and examined the efficacy of a peer counseling model. The structured intervention included encouragement to maintain interpersonal relationships, to make positive plans for the future, to query the medical staff regarding treatments, side effects, and sexual outcomes, and to maintain normal routines. These interventions were delivered in three telephone contacts (one pre-treatment and at 5 and 10 weeks post-treatment) and with provision of a booklet and audiotape description of the coping strategies at the pre-treatment hospital visit. Two former cancer patients, who were also trained as social workers, were the peer counselors. Thirty-two women participated. Measures assessed emotional distress and coping strategies. Analyses indicated no differences between groups from pre- to post-treatment.

There are three experimental studies. Two reports included women with breast cancer. Davis (1986) reported a small scale outcome study comparing two behavior therapies (biofeedback along with progressive relaxation training versus cognitive behavior therapy and progressive relaxation training) with a no treatment control. Twenty-five women recently treated for early stage breast cancer participated. Findings indicated a significant reduction with time in anxiety for all women but no differential improvement for the intervention subjects. Christensen (1983) reported on a focused intervention for adjustment difficulties of mastectomy patients and their partners. The program included discussion of the history of the relationship, readings and discussions of the emotional and sexual aspects of mastectomy, disclosure of feelings and fantasies of the self and the spouse and other exercises (communication training, role playing) to facilitate confronting and solving problems. The format was conjoint for 4 weekly sessions. Twenty women treated from 2 to 3 months previously participated. Analyses indicated the intervention had modest effects in reducing distress for the breast cancer patients, but significant improvements for the couple occurred in sexual satisfaction.

The largest and most comprehensive investigation was conducted by Fawzy and colleagues (1990 a and b) and attempted to reduce distress and enhance immune functioning in newly diagnosed melanoma patients. A structured group support intervention was offered which included health education, illness-related problem solving, relaxation training and group support. The format was weekly group treatment for six sessions. Eighty patients (53 percent female) with early stage melanoma participated and were randomized to intervention or control conditions. The post-treatment analyses indicated that the intervention subjects reported significantly more vigor, but there were no other emotional distress differences. By six months, emotional distress had improved for the intervention subjects with significantly lower depression, confusion, and fatigue, and higher vigor. Coping data indicated that the intervention subjects reported significantly more use of active-behavioral strategies by treatment's end, a pattern which continued with the addition of active-cognitive strategies by six months. Regarding the immunologic findings, at six months there was a significant difference in groups with better immunologic status in the intervention subjects.

While there are limitations to these investigations, the quasi-experimental designs suggested that broad-based interventions produced few gains in psychological or behavioral outcomes, but significant improvement was found in sexual functioning. The rapid emotional improvement which occurs following cancer treatment may have contributed to the findings of no differential outcome or only modest improvement in emotional distress. However, follow up data suggested some consolidation of intervention effects across time (upwards of 6 months post-treatment), with lowered emotional distress and/or enhanced coping coupled with confirming immunologic outcomes. Finally, these gains are all the more impressive by their achievement with brief therapy (eg. 10 therapy hours).

Treatment

A certain component of the emotional distress occurring at diagnosis is the anticipation of undergoing difficult treatment(s). Current therapies include surgery, radiotherapy and treatment with radioactive substances, chemotherapy, hormonal therapy, immunotherapy and combination regimens and procedures (eg. bone marrow transplantation, intraoperative radiotherapy). Some patients also need difficult diagnostic or treatment monitoring procedures (eg. bone marrow aspirations) and all treatments are preceded and followed by physical examinations, tumor surveys, and/or laboratory studies. Thus, cancer treatments represent significant stressors and the data are consistent in their portrayal of more distress (particularly fear and anxiety), slower rates of emotional recovery and, perhaps, additional behavioral difficulties (eg. panic attacks) than are found with healthy individuals also undergoing medical treatment (eg. hysterectomy, cholecystectomy, hernia repair) for benign conditions. Despite this fact, the crisis level of emotional distress at diagnosis lessens during treatment initiation, continuance, and early recovery (ie. 2 to 12 months post-treatment; Andersen et al., 1989b; Bloom, 1987; Devlen et al., 1987). This lowering of emotional distress over time is found even for patients undergoing radical treatment requiring major adjustments (eg. radical neck dissection with laryngectomy; Manuel et al., 1987).

There have been few investigations of cancer surgery, but there are numerous descriptive and intervention studies of the reactions of healthy individuals undergoing surgery for benign conditions. The latter studies are consistent in their portrayal of (a) high levels of self-reported pre-operative anxiety predictive of lowered post-operative anxiety and (b) post-operative anxiety predictive of recovery (eg. time out of bed, pain reports). What may distinguish cancer surgery patients are higher overall levels of distress and slower rates of emotional recovery. Gottesman and Lewis (1982) found greater and more lasting feelings of crisis and helplessness among cancer patients in comparison to benign surgery patients for as long as two months following discharge. Considering these data, findings on the interaction patterns of physicians and cancer patients on morning surgical rounds is disturbing. Blanchard and colleagues (1987) found attending physicians on a cancer unit to be less likely to be supportive and address patients' needs than physicians treating general medical patients. The heavier volume and more seriously ill patients common to cancer units might be sources for this unfortunate relationship. Related findings indicate that oncology nurses might find their job significantly more stressful than other assignments (eg. cardiac, intensive care, or operating room nursing; Stewart *et al.*, 1982).

At least 350,000 individuals receive radiation therapy each year. Clinical descriptions have noted patient's fears (eg, being burned, hair loss, sterility); such outcomes do occur, but they are site and dosage dependent. To understand radiation fears, the surgical anxiety studies already described above have been a paradigm. Here, again, high levels of anticipatory anxiety are found, but if interventions to reduce distress are not conducted, heightened post-treatment anxiety is also found (Andersen *et al.*, 1984; Andersen and Tewfik, 1985) and might be maintained for as long as three months post therapy, particularly when treatment symptoms (eg. diarrhea, fatigue) linger (King *et al.*, 1985). When acute side effects resolve (usually by 12 months post-treatment), there appears to be no higher incidence of emotional difficulties for radiotherapy patients than for surgery patients (Hughson *et al.*, 1987).

Of all the treatment modalities, the greatest progress has been in the understanding of psychological reactions to chemotherapy, particularly the side effects of nausea and vomiting. Research has also targeted the development of interventions to reduce anxiety and determine individual (ie. high pre-treatment anxiety or general distress, severity of post-treatment vomiting in the early cycles, age) and situational (ie. more emetogenic regimens, higher dosages or greater amounts of chemotherapy) differences that place patients at risk (see Carey and Burish, 1988 for a review). With continued psychological research, improvement in antiemetic drugs and efforts to reduce drug toxicity, many of these gastrointestinal effects might be reduced if not eliminated.

Finally, psychological and behavioral data have been (and should continue to be) important to patients and physicians alike for making choices among comparable curative treatments. Treatments that result in less disruption often become 'standard' treatment. The most obvious example of the importance of psychological data influencing cancer treatments was that documenting the more positive (ie. lower psychological distress, fewer sexual difficulties) outcomes for women treated with breast saving (segmental mastectomy with adjuvant radiotherapy) procedures rather than modified radical mastectomy.

There have been psychological efforts to assist women during and immediately following cancer treatment. Cain *et al.* (1986) compared individual and group therapy formats. The intervention had eight components including discussion of the causes of cancer at diagnosis, impact of the treatment(s) on body image and sexuality, relaxation training, emphasis on good dietary and exercise patterns, dealing with communication difficulties with medical staff and friends/family and setting goals for the future to cope with uncertainty and fears of recurrence. The eight session program was conducted during individual sessions in the hospital or the women's home or in weekly groups of 4–6 patients carried out at the hospital. Seventy-two women with gynecologic cancer completed the study. Outcome measures were administered pre- and post-treatment and at a 6-month follow up. Post-treatment analyses indicated all groups improved with time; however, anxiety was significantly lower for the individual therapy subjects only. Gains for the intervention subjects were more impressive at 6-month follow up; there were no differences between the intervention formats, but intervention groups reported less depression and anxiety and better psychosocial adjustment (including health perspectives, sexual function and use of leisure time) than the no treatment control group. Thus, the brief intervention, delivered either in individual or groups formats, appeared to be immediately effective, with gains enhanced during the early recovery months.

Several papers by Maguire and colleagues (eg. Maguire, *et al.*, 1985) describe the outcomes following individual counselling for women with breast cancer in the UK. A nurse specialist provided an intervention to restore mobility to the affected arm through movement exercises, to facilitate adjustment to the scar and breast loss by disclosing feelings, and to encourage the return to social activities and employment. The format was individual and conducted in the hospital pre-surgery and in the patient's home. One hundred and fifty-two women treated with modified radical mastectomy and node dissection participated. Physical outcomes appeared to be better for the counselled women, with fewer reporting problems with swelling or pain. Also, psychological responses to breast loss were judged to be better. There were fewer difficulties when returning to housework and/or employment, and there were fewer problems with social relationships for the counselled women. There were significantly more episodes and more severe episodes of anxiety or depression (eg. 3 percent vs. 19 percent of the intervention and control groups, respectively) in the control group. Finally, marital and sexual adjustment was also better for the counselled women.

Telch and Telch (1986) compared the effectiveness of coping skills instruction with supportive therapy for a heterogeneous sample of cancer patients on follow up. A novel aspect was that potential subjects were screened and only those with "clear evidence of psychological distress" were eligible. Both interventions were offered in a group format. The coping skills instruction taught cognitive, behavioral and affective coping strategies and included goal setting, self monitoring and role playing. Relaxation training and stress management skills were also included and patients provided ratings of their home practice. The group support intervention provided an environment for patients to discuss concerns but there was no specific agenda. Each group met for six weeks. Forty-one cancer patients completed the study; 66 percent of the sample was female. Analyses for the emotional distress data indicated that the coping skills group improved significantly across all measures, the group support group improved on the anxiety and depression only, but the no treatment control worsened and reported significantly more mood distress.

In summary, these data attest to the signficantly greater distress which occurs when patients are still in the midst of treatment. Unlike the weaker effects at post-treatment for patients when they have concluded treatment, more impressive gains were found when patients are in the midst of treatment and the effects are stronger with continued follow up. Again, these effects were achieved with very brief interventions.

Recovery

The most important cancer endpoints have been treatment response rates, length of disease-free interval, and survival. Yet as the prognosis for some sites has improved, there has been increased attention paid to the quality of life following treatment. For the cured cancer patient (ie. typically referring to individuals surviving at least five years, as the probability of late recurrence declines significantly after that time for most sites), it has been suggested that there are two broad classes of stressors (Cella and Tross, 1986). The first includes residual sequelae, including lingering emotional distress from the trauma of diagnosis, treatment, and, more generally, life threat (perhaps this reaction is analogous to that of post-traumatic stress disorder). The second class of stressors includes continuing sequelae, including confrontation with the changes to the person's premorbid life (eg. loss of speech following laryngectomy) and adjustment requiring new behaviors/emotions and/or coping with losses (eg. a sexual relationship that does not include intercourse).

The earliest writings (from the 1950s to the 1980s) suggested that the psychological trajectory was, at best, difficult with somatic problems, psychological distress, impaired relationships, preoccupation with death and/or general life disruption, such as reduced employment or career opportunities (eg. Bard and Sutherland, 1952; Schonfield, 1972). Many of these pioneering reports were clinical and, in general, uncontrolled on disease variables now recognized as moderators of adjustment. By the end of this same period, cancer had become more public, more survivable and clinical trials were able to examine treatment toxicity (ie. side effects) following the establishment of effectiveness. These important changes account, in part, for the more positive findings presently emerging in the study of long-term adjustment.

If the disease is controlled and recovery from treatment proceeds unimpaired, longitudinal data indicate that, by one year post-treatment the severe distress of diagnosis will have dissipated and emotions will have stabilized. The first longitudinal studies conducted in the United Kingdom for breast cancer patients indicated that by 12 (Maguire *et al.*, 1978) and 24 months (Morris, *et al.*, 1977) approximately 20 percent of the patients had problems with moderate to severe depression in comparison to 8 percent of benign disease comparison subjects. However, more recent controlled longitudinal studies of breast (Bloom, 1987; Vinokur *et al.*, 1989) and gynecologic (Anderson *et al.*, 1989b) patients conducted in the United States and replicated by data from the Netherlands (de Haes *et al.*, 1986) have indicated no differences between the levels of emotional distress of women with cancer and either benign disease or healthy comparison subjects. Similar declines and lowered levels of distress have been found in retrospective (Cella and Tross, 1986) and longitudinal (Devlen *et al.*, 1987) studies of Hodgkin's disease and non-Hodgkin's lymphoma patients.

The consistency of findings for the studies conducted during the 1980s is important because it represents replications across site and, to some degree, treatment toxicity. For cancer patients with previous psychiatric histories, the rates of depression following treatment would be higher than for patients without this risk factor. A variety of individuals with a psychiatric history, however, report greater distress, poorer adjustment and so forth following a medical event than patients without a psychiatric history (eg. O'Hara *et al.*, 1984). In sum, there is no evidence suggesting that cancer precipitates additional or more severe psychiatric episodes than would otherwise occur.

All women with solid tumors (approximately 85 percent of adult patients) are vulnerable to sexual dysfunction. Across sites, estimates range from 10 percent (eg. breast cancer patients treated with lumpectomy; Steinberg *et al.*, 1985) to 70–90 percent (eg. women with vulva cancer treated with modified radical vulvectomy), with the distribution skewed toward greater levels of disruption. Among the hematologic malignancies, like Hodgkin's Disease, estimates are in the range of 20 percent. Although the majority of the data comes from small sample retrospective reports (see Andersen, 1985, for a discussion), the data within sites have been consistent and convincing in their suggestion of disease and treatment factors as the etiologic bases for these problems. Controlled longitudinal studies of breast cancer patients (Maguire *et al.*, 1978; Morris *et al.*, 1977) and gynecologic cancer patients (Andersen *et al.*, 1989a) have indicated that if sexual problems develop, they do so as soon as intercourse resumes and, if untreated, they are unlikely to be resolved.

The high incidence of sexual and fertility disruption has, in part, been the reason for the concern over marital disruption among adult cancer patients. For example, an early clinical study of women receiving radical mastectomy noted the realistic feelings of body disfigurement that both the women and spouses would feel, prompting sexual retreat, emotional estrangement, and, not surprisingly, marital disruption (Bard and Sutherland, 1952). Other concerns over the marriage originate from analyses of the interpersonal relationships, per se, of cancer patients (Wortman and Dunkel-Schetter, 1979). Despite the emotional distress and, for some, accompanying sexual disruption that couples experience, data from retrospective studies with comparison groups (Cella and Tross, 1986) and from the controlled longitudinal studies previously discussed indicate that most marriages remain intact and satisfactory. These data are consistent with prospective studies showing that, when health problems arise for newly married couples, they are not among those problems precipitant to divorce (Bentler and Newcomb, 1978).

Data on the interpersonal relationships of cancer patients suggest that, in general, satisfaction predominates. The majority of relationships remain intact, satisfactory, and, on occasion, stronger, as found in data from single assessment (Baider and Sarell, 1984; Lichtman and Taylor, 1986; Meyerowitz *et al.*, 1983) and longitudinal (Neuling and Winefield, 1988) studies. When problems do occur, they include estrangement and distress which were originally hypothesized for the majority of patients (Wortman and Dunkel-Schetter, 1979). In addition, the cancer experience is stressful for those closest to the patient and the kin's distress may approach that of the patient's (Cassileth *et al.*, 1985). Further, in young families when the wife/mother has cancer and there are young children are in the home, such families may be at heightened risk (Vess, *et al.* 1985).

Recurrence and Death

Recurrence is devastating; the magnitude of distress is even greater than that found with the initial diagnosis (Thompson *et al.*, 1992), and studies contrasting cancer patients showing no evidence of disease with those receiving palliative treatment (eg. Cassileth *et al.*, 1985) have reported the greatest distress for those with disseminated disease (Bloom, 1987). Difficult decisions (eg. beginning a regimen that offers little chance for cure and has side effects vs. no treatment) are made in a context of extreme emotional distress and physical debilitation.

At this time of significant emotional turmoil and physical difficulty, psychological interventions appear to enhance the quality of life. In 1979 Ferlic, Goldman, and Kennedy published the first randomized intervention study with cancer patients. An interdisciplinary, crisis intervention program was offered which included patient education (introduction to the hospital, cancer as a disease, cancer treatments, etc.), presentations by medical team members (physician, nurse, social worker, chaplain, dietician) and supportive group therapy (including topics of emotional distress, coping, sexuality, strain on family/social relationships, etc.). The format was group meetings for six sessions. Sixty adults (50 percent female) with 'advanced' cancer participated. Patients were at "varying stages of their cancer treatment" with a mean of seven weeks since diagnosis. A six month follow up was attempted. However, mortality (20 percent of the intervention and 33 percent of the controls died) and insufficient questionnaire returns (30 percent and 60 percent for control and treatment, respectively) precluded proper data analysis. Nevertheless the intervention group showed improvement in adjustment across all treatment areas, whereas the controls improved in three, relationship strength, cancer information and death perceptions. Also, the self concept score for the intervention group significantly increased, whereas that for the control group significantly decreased.

Several papers have described the outcomes of the group support intervention for women with breast cancer of Spiegel, Bloom and colleagues (Spiegel *et al.*, 1981; Spiegel and Bloom, 1983). Women were randomized to no treatment or a group treatment intervention which included discussion of death and dying, family problems, communication problems with physicians and living fully in the context of a terminal illness. The intervention subjects were also randomized a second time to two conditions: no additional treatments or self hypnosis for pain problems (Spiegel and Bloom, 1983), which was incorporated into the support group format. All intervention groups met for weekly meetings for one year, for a total of 75 therapy hours. At the end of the first year the groups formally ended, but members could continue to meet as they wished or were able; some groups lasted for an additional two years. Eighty-six women, 50 intervention and 36 no treatment control, with metastic breast cancer, participated. Following random assignment, there was subject loss (eg. refusal, too weak, death) with the study beginning with 34 intervention and 24 control participants, although the survival data are reported for the original sample of 86. Analyses indicated that the intervention group reported significantly fewer phobic responses and lower anxiety, fatigue and confusion and higher vigor than the controls. These differences were evident at all assessments but the magnitude increased from 4 to 12 months. There was also a significant decrease in the use of maladaptive coping responses by the intervention group. Regarding the findings from the hypnosis substudy, women receiving hypnosis within the group support intervention reported no change in their pain sensations during the year, while pain sensations significantly increased for the other women in group support who did not receive hypnosis. Similar findings were reported for pain suffering; a slight decrease for the women who also received hypnosis and a significant increase in suffering for the remaining intervention women. It is important to note, however, that pain sensation scores for both groups were significantly lower than those for the no intervention controls, suggesting that the hypnosis component provided an additive analgesic effect to other group treatment components. The most startling data from this project was reported in a survival analysis described at the beginning of the chapter. A variety of follow up analyses, controlling for initial disease stage, days of radiotherapy, or use or androgen or steroid treatments were conducted and all indicated the same survival differences favoring the intervention participants.

CONCLUSION

Significant progress has been made in understanding the psychological and behavioral aspects of cancer in women. Contributions are significant in the areas of prevention and control of breast cancer, but there has been less research on other prevalent cancer sites. Research on smoking prevention and cessation has the potential to have an impact on the factor responsible for 30 percent of all cancer deaths and will be important for women in view of their increasing lung cancer rates.

More is known about the psychological processes and reactions to the diagnosis and treatment of cancer than is known about any other chronic illness. Although most is known about the adjustment of breast cancer patients (see Glanz and Lerman, in press, for a review), other disease sites, such as gynecologic, are being studied more. Future research needs to test the generalizability of these descriptive data and formulate general principles of adjustment to illness. While providing estimates of the magnitude of quality of life problems, these data can be used for models which predict which women might be at greatest risk for adjustment difficulties (see Andersen, in press for a discussion). The latter is an important step toward designing interventions tailored to the difficulties and circumstances of women with cancer.

A growing literature on the use of psychological interventions to improve the quality of life for women with cancer also exists. The effectiveness of these interventions is robust, as they have reduced distress and enhanced the quality of life of many cancer patients differing in disease stage as well as disease site. Despite the challenges of studying these patients, well controlled investigations have been conducted. Improvements in emotional distress are found at the end of the interventions and gains are as continued at follow up. In addition, change in other areas; self esteem/concept, death perceptions, life satisfaction, and/or locus of control, have been found. Importantly for quality of life, psychological interventions could also lower or stabilize pain reports. The positive outcomes for terminal patients are notable considering their worsening pain and/or increasing debilitation. Unlike the other studies, interventions for terminal patients were intensive and lengthy, such as "several sessions," "until death," or at least 75 hours.

While there appear to be unique intervention components for different phases in the disease, there are some commonalities. Therapy components have included: an *emotionally supportive context* to address fears and anxieties about the disease, *information about the disease and treatment, behavioral coping strategies, cognitive coping strategies,* and *relaxation training* to lower 'arousal' and/or enhance one's sense of control. The descriptive data also highlight the need for *focused interventions* for sexual functioning, particularly those treated for gynecologic or breast cancer and the intervention studies attest to the effectiveness of this specific component. These components appear more important to the outcome than procedural variations. For example, therapy format, such as individual or group, appears to have little impact. Also, there were null findings for (group) interventions that included no structured content, suggesting that group support alone is insufficient to produce any measurable benefit.

How do psychological interventions achieve these effects? In large measure, the psychologic mechanisms may not be different from those operating in interventions designed for coping with other stressors. That is, confronting a traumatic stressor with positive cognitive states, active behavioral strategies and, eventually, lowered emotional distress may enhance one's sense of self efficacy, feelings of control and provide realistic appraisals of stresses of the disease or treatment process. Similarly for sexual interventions, information provides realistic expectations for sexuality and specific strategies to manage sexual activity when it is difficult. That the interventions produce more than situational improvement and may alter an individual's longer term adjustment processes is suggested by the data indicating that adjustment gains continue (and often increase) during the first post-treatment year. Immediate and longer term psychologic changes may, in turn, increase the likelihood of changes in behavioral mechanisms, such as increasing the likelihood of adaptive health behaviors (eg. complying with medical therapy; improving diet, exercise, etc.), to improve mental health directly, 'adjustment' and, possibly, medical outcomes. These data indicate that increasingly, issues of quality of life are being raised and positive results have been achieved by behavioral sciences. But as with most issues, further commitment and action is needed.

FURTHER READING

Andersen, B.L. (Ed.) (1986). *Women with cancer: Psychological perspectives*. New York: Springer-Verlag.
Holland, J.C. and Rowland, J.H. (Eds.) (1989). *Handbook of psycho-oncology: Psychological care of patient with cancer*. New York: Oxford University Press.

7

WOMEN AND HIV/AIDS: CHALLENGING A GROWING THREAT

MICHELE GOLDSCHMIDT AND
LYDIA TEMOSHOK

*Henry M. Jackson Foundation for the Advancement of Military Medicine,
1 Taft Court, Suite 250, Rockville, Maryland 20850, USA*

GEORGE R. BROWN

*Wilford Hall Medical Center, Lackland Air Force Base, San Antonio,
Texas 78235, USA*

The World Health Organization (WHO), 1991, November 11) estimates that three quarters of the 8–10 million people infected with HIV worldwide have been infected through heterosexual contact. In central Africa, where more than half of those infected live, heterosexual contact has been the predominant mode of transmission since the pandemic began. The results have been devastating. As of November, 1991, the WHO reported that HIV disease is split nearly equally between more than 6 million men and women and has affected an estimated 900,000 children. The picture is being repeated in India, Latin America and Southeast Asia (*South*, 1991).

In North America and Western Europe, where the primary modes of transmission have been homosexual and bisexual contact and intravenous drug abuse (IVDA), the threat posed by 'straight sex' has been largely denied by society until recently. The *International Conference on the Implications of AIDS for Mothers and Children*, held in

Mandatory disclaimer
The opinions or assertions contained herein are the private views of the authors and are not to be construed as official or as reflecting the views of the Henry M. Jackson Foundation for the Advancement of Military Medicine or the Department of Defense.

Paris, France, November 27–30, 1989 underscored the problem in Western Europe and appealed for aggressive strategies to promote and protect the health of families (*World Health*, 1990). One year later, the First National Conference on Women and HIV was held in Washington, DC (December 12–13, 1990) to focus attention on the growing problem in the United States (National Institute for Allergy and Infectious Diseases [NIAID] & Centers for Disease Control [CDC], 1991). As a result of these meetings, popular articles began to appear in the US, increasing the public's awareness. a pivotal point came when Earvin 'Magic' Johnson, a US sports hero, announced his own infection in November, 1991, resulting in unprecedented media coverage.

Of the total number of AIDS cases in the US, less than 6 percent are reportedly attributable to heterosexual transmission. However, the US CDC (1990; 1991) reported that the proportion jumped 41 percent between October, 1990 and October, 1991, faster than any other category. Over half of those cases were related to sex with a drug abusing partner; 22 percent more traced their origins to a country where heterosexual contact is the most likely mode of transmission. These risks have been clearly identified; however, 22 percent of the cases did not report any behaviors that had put them at risk, up from 16 percent just the year before. Further, HIV is spreading to rural areas and small to medium-sized cities, previously characterized by their low prevalences (Ellerbrock *et al.*, 1991). In a highly mobile society such as the US, the numbers of infected individuals are expected to increase.

The rise in heterosexually acquired infections has serious implications for women. Women are the fastest growing group infected with HIV. In the US, women make up over 12 percent of the total numbers of adult/adolescent AIDS cases reported to the CDC, up from 9.7 percent in 1990 and 8.8 in 1989 (CDC, 1989; 1990; 1991). Heterosexual transmission accounts for at least 34 percent of the cases of AIDS in women in the US (CDC, 1991) and 26 percent in Europe (Oxtoby, 1991). Only intravenous drug abuse reportedly accounts for more cases (51 percent in the US and 56 percent in Europe) and the gap is closing. Brown and Rundell (1990) reported that heterosexual transmission is the rule in infected female military medical beneficiaries and Carpenter *et al.* (1991) reported that heterosexual contact has been the dominant mode of transmission in their population of HIV infected women in the state of Rhode Island since the latter part of 1990.

Although risk factors are similar, epidemiologic evidence points to gender differences in how HIV is acquired. In a landmark study using CDC data through the end of 1986, Guinan and Hardy (1987a) found that of 456 adults infected heterosexually, 84 percent were female. Compared to HIV infected men, women were more than four times as likely to have been infected heterosexually (Guinan and Hardy, 1987b). The authors found this to be the only risk category where women outnumbered men. In their study of discordant (positive-negative) couples, Padian, Shiboski and Jewell (1991) recently supported the evidence that men may transmit HIV more efficiently than women. They found that women were 17.5 times more likely to become infected than men (other factors being held constant). Although Padian *et al.* acknowledged the usual limitations due to subjects' recall of risk histories, the differences could not be explained by number of exposures or types of risk behaviors. Being the receptive sexual partner (whether heterosexual or homosexual) appears to play a role in transmission (Chin, 1990).

In central Africa, where the prevalence rates are equal, the risks for HIV to men may be higher than in the US because of a higher rate of sexually transmitted diseases (STDs). Piot and Laga (1989) theorized that the presence of mucosal lesions from other STDs facilitates transmission of HIV. Indeed, genital ulcer disease is a risk factor in both the US and in Africa (Chirgwin *et al.*, 1991), but to a far greater extent in Africa.

Eighty-five percent of women with AIDS reported to the CDC in December, 1990 were of reproductive age (15–44 years) (Ellerbrock *et al.*, 1991). Therefore, it is not surprising that the rising trend in the numbers of cases of AIDS in children parallels that of women, increasing 26 percent between 1990 and 1991 (CDC, 1990; 1991). More than 80 percent of infected children in the US and 70 per cent in Europe acquired the disease perinatally (CDC, 1990, December; Oxtoby, 1991). Half of these cases were the result of drug abuse by the mother and 30 percent linked (heterosexually) to the male partner (Oxtoby, 1991). As other routes of transmission become less important (eg. blood transfusions), it is expected that these proportions will increase also.

Ethnic minority women represent the highest proportion of women infected with HIV in the US. Although African-American and Latina women make up 19 percent of the female population, they represent 73 percent of AIDS cases in women (CDC, 1991). Even though the numbers of cases are increasing for all women, the new cases in minority women are increasing disproportionately fast. Ellerbrock *et al.* (1991) found that Latina and African-American women had cumulative incidence rates 8 and 13 times, respectively, that for white women. Chu, Buehler and Berkelman (1990) reported that African-American women were nine times more likely to die of AIDS than white women (10.3 versus 1.2 per 100,000). HIV/AIDS is the leading cause of death among African-American women aged 15–44 in New York and New Jersey and among women in major cities throughout central Africa and Western Europe (Chu *et al.*, 1990; WHO, 1990).

Despite these statistics and the fact that AIDS cases have been described in women since 1981, until very recently, policymakers and researchers have largely ignored women as victims of HIV. National attention first focused on women's concerns in December, 1990 at the Washington meeting. Other than case reports and anecdotes, the little data that existed were considered 'soft' (Chavkin *et al.*, 1991) and lacked gender-specific research findings from large-scale prospective studies (Miller *et al.*, 1990). A comprehensive literature review of three leading psychiatry journals in the US from 1985 to 1991 revealed 31 studies examining psychosocial aspects of HIV infection in 2,438 individuals, only 13 of whom were women (Nakajima and Rubin, 1991).

At the same time, it is important to note that women have never been ignored completely. Noteworthy exceptions to the 'soft' data include two prospective studies: a study on the psychiatric morbidity and biopsychosocial aspects of HIV in women conducted by one of us (Brown) and colleagues since 1987 (Brown and Rundell, 1990; Brown and Rundell, in press) and a study on the demography, natural history, clinical manifestations and societal impact of HIV infection on women from 1986 through 1990 by Carpenter *et al.* (1991). Unfortunately, in other studies, women have been seen as 'vehicles of transmission' of the disease to men via the commercial sex industry (Campbell, 1990) and intravenous drug abuse (Des Jarlais *et al.*, 1990) and to their children (Andiman and Modlin, 1991). Much of the early research on women and HIV came from data collected on pregnant women by researchers trying to understand and prevent perinatal transmission.

Nevertheless, for the most part, women have been, as Rosser (1991, p. 231) pointed out, the "missing persons" in the US HIV/AIDS epidemic. In this chapter, we attempt to redress this gender imbalance. First, we present a summary of the biological and clinical picture of HIV infection in women. Next, we discuss the psychosocial impact of HIV/AIDS on women's lives. Finally, we review the recent directions taken by the research community to focus attention on women and HIV.

BIOLOGICAL AND CLINICAL MANIFESTATIONS

HIV is a progressive disease, characterized by the destruction of the immune system and with it, the body's ability to fight infections. The human immunodeficiency virus (type 1) attacks and depletes a specific set of white blood cells known as CD4 (T4 or helper T) lymphocytes (Redfield and Burke, 1988). The CD4 cells are crucial in mediating cellular immunity. Their loss impairs the body's ability to combat viruses, bacteria, fungi and parasites, leaving it vulnerable to a host of infections. In a defenseless system, these opportunistic infections (OIs) are deadly. Because it is expensive and time-consuming to isolate the virus itself, the presence of HIV is indirectly determined by testing for antibodies created against viral proteins. The tests are known as the ELISA (enzyme-linked immunoabsorbent assay) for the initial screening and Western Blot for confirmation of positive ELISA tests. They have a combined sensitivity and specificity of better than 99 percent and have been widely available since 1985.

The time period from infection to AIDS, the end-stage of HIV disease, may be at least 10 years. During this time, HIV infected persons may be entirely asymptomatic (but infectious), or present with viermia (influenze-like symptoms caused by the body's initial response to the virus), or non-specific complaints such as fatigue (Redfield *et al.*, 1986). In 1981, in order to isolate the cause of the mysterious syndrome that manifested itself as a cluster of rare diseases in persons who became severely immunocompromised, the CDC adopted a strict epidemiological-surveillance definition for AIDS (Redfield and Burke, 1988). People were said to have AIDS if they developed Kaposi's sarcoma (a rare skin cancer) or any of a few designated OIs (especially *Pneumocystis carinii* pneumonia [PCP]). By 1984, research had identified HIV as the cause of AIDS, but also that persons with AIDS represented only the tip of the iceberg. The CDC's (1987) revised definition added other OIs, but remained narrowly focused on the end-stage of HIV disease.

In order to begin early, effective treatment for HIV infected individuals, Redfield *et al.* (1986) developed a system to classify seropositive individuals (identified via routine screening) by degree of immune dysfunction. Individuals classified as Stage 0 have been potentially exposed to HIV by a carrier but have not seroconverted. Infected individuals progress from Stage 1 (recently seroconverted; CD4 cells $> 500/mm^3$) to Stage 6 (equivalent to the most recent CDC definition of AIDS [effective April, 1992]; CD4 cells $\leqslant 200/mm^3$). The full spectrum of conditions which can develop when the immune system is weakened has not been described, although about a dozen diseases predominate. Table 7.1 lists the most common or virulent infections in HIV infected persons. Gynecological infections, often the first sign of HIV in women, must be added to this list. Table 7.2 lists the most common medical conditions among HIV infected women. The primary clinical difference between men and women is in the

TABLE 7.1

Most Common HIV-related Infections in the US (Source: Redfield and Burke, 1988).

Cryptosporidiosis
Cryptococcosis
Cytomegalovirus
Herpes simplex
Histoplasmosis
Legionella
Leukoplakia (Oral, hairy)
Molluscum Contagiosum
Pneumocystis carinii pneumonia (PCP)
Salmonella
Syphilis, secondary
Thrush (Oral Candidiasis)
Toxoplasmosis
Tuberculosis

TABLE 7.2

Most Common Medical Conditions among HIV Infected Women (Source: Denenberg, 1990).

Abnormal Pap Smears
Candida esophagitis
Candida vaginitis
Human papilloma virus infection (HPV)
Neoplasia of the cervix, vagina and vulva
Pelvic Inflammatory Disease (PID)
Streptococcus pneumoniae

number of specific OIs experienced. Women suffer more frequently from *Candida* and herpes simplex infections (Minkoff and DeHovitz, 1991) and less frequently from Kaposi's sarcoma (Beral *et al.*, 1990). Additionally, HIV infected women who are intravenous drug abusers (IVDAs) have more cervical dysplasia and neoplasms than women infected heterosexually, a factor believed to be linked to total number of sexual partners (Carpenter *et al.*, 1991).

Antiretroviral therapy is essentially the same for men and non-pregnant women (NIAID, CDC, 1991), although Minkoff and De Hovitz (1991) caution against dismissing the possibility of a gender effect in pharmacokinetics due to the lack of definitive data. The two drugs approved by the Food and Drug Administration (FDA) are zidovudine (formerly AZT) and most recently dideoxyinosine (ddI). The CDC recommends that one of these drugs be used when an individual's CD4 cell count drops below 500/mm^3. Recent efforts to delay the onset of OIs have met with considerable success and are intensifying (Cotton, 1991).

Early drug prophylaxis and therapies failed to extend the lives of persons with AIDS because little was known about how to treat OIs. Research devoted to this area was inadequate because antiretroviral research was more "glamorous" (Cotton, 1991, p. 1476). Some of the impetus to develop better drugs and treatment methods came from activist groups who consult with researchers in developing clinical trials. Recent advances are changing the clinical picture, slowing down the progression to AIDS and prolonging lives even when cell counts are very low ($>50/mm^3$). A major drawback of these therapies is that they do not attack malignancies. To detect neoplasms in women, Carpenter *et al.* (1991) recommend frequent cervico-vaginal cytologic studies, semi-annually for IVDAs and annually for women infected heterosexually.

There is sufficient evidence to suggest that the course of HIV infection in women given early, effective and consistent treatment in a socially well-supported environment, is no more rapid and may be less virulent than in men (Carpenter *et al.*, 1991). Unfortunately, the majority of women with HIV are diagnosed late in the course of their disease. Because gynecological conditions are common in women with or without HIV, a woman's health care provider may be the first point of contact for women at risk for infection. However, because the risks for HIV to women have not been the focus of educational campaigns, policymaking and research, health care providers may neglect to consider HIV as an underlying cause of the infections. Prior to the CDC's latest revised definition for AIDS, Carpenter *et al.* (1991) suggested that the combination of recurrent vaginal candidiasis *and* a CD4 count of $\leqslant 200/mm^3$ warrants a diagnosis of AIDS in HIV positive women.

Many in the medical community have needed coaxing to treat women infected with HIV actively. Some of the impetus came from within the fields of obstetrics/gynecology and midwifery. Although primarily involved with pregnant women, Minkoff (1987) and his colleagues, in particular, have done much to educate and persuade health care providers to counsel, screen and care for all women at risk. Recognizing the growing risks to women from heterosexual transmission, Minkoff and Landesman (1988) argued for offering routine HIV testing to all pregnant women. The authors observed that when HIV entered the heterosexual community, it became more difficult to determine who was at risk. Additionally, as we noted, the benefits of early clinical intervention are now clearly recognized. Moreover, early intervention can foster changes in behavior and prevent transmission. These benefits strengthen the views of those (eg. Redfield and Burke, 1988) who support offering screening for HIV as a standard routine in health care.

In another persuasive article, Minkoff and Moreno (1990) countered the CDC's (1989) position that drug prophylaxis in pregnant women with low CD4 cell counts should begin after pregnancy. To protect themselves against lawsuits resulting from potential fetal injury, drug companies have traditionally excluded pregnant women from participating in clinical trials. As a result, insufficient data exist to determine whether prophylactic agents are indeed teratogenic (or abortifacient) to the fetus, although preliminary reports suggest they are not (Minkoff and Feinkind, 1989). On the other hand, there is some evidence to suggest that pregnancy, itself a cause of immune changes, may accelerate the progress of HIV disease in women who are already in the late stages of HIV infection (see eg. Fox, 1991). Further, several studies have documented higher rates of infection or mortality in infants born to mothers in late stage disease in Africa (Ryder *et al.*, 1989), or whose mothers died within one year of pregnancy in the US (Koonin *et al.*, 1989). Minkoff and Moreno contend that withholding information about all available treatment options seriously impairs the physician-patient relationship and interferes with a woman's autonomy. Thus, they argue, it is prudent to offer each woman the opportunity to decide whether drug prophylaxis during pregnancy is appropriate for her.

THE PSYCHOSOCIAL IMPACT OF HIV/AIDS ON WOMEN

"Honey", he said, "I have HIV."

With those few words, a woman shares with him the threat of a potentially fatal disease that remains underscored by lingering stigma and social isolation. She feels anger, then sorrow at the prospect of her own death and guilt at the threat to her present – and future – children. When the numbing shock subsides, she may get tested, and then agonize a little more as she waits for the results. Alternatively, she may not want to know her serostatus; if she is poor, she may feel she has no control over her situation and that little will be gained by knowing. She worries about the loss of economic support and the pressures of mounting health care bills. Chances are, she won't leave him. She cares for him throughout his illness and death. She figures out ways to provide for her children should she, too, become disabled; and arranges custody for them should she die. She must also deal with the behaviors that had placed the family at risk, if indeed she knows what they are. Moreover, she tries to educate her family and friends to prevent this from happening to them.

"Honey", she said, "I have HIV."

If he tests negative, he may leave her. Why should he risk his health and sexual future on a woman who may give him a fatal disease? If he tests positive, he may blame her for giving it to him (although it is far more likely to have been the other way around) and still leave her – in anger. Unlike him, she often faces HIV alone. Her gynecologist may not know how to treat her, or how to enroll her in the clinical trials designed to provide some answers. The HIV/AIDS clinic may not deal with her gynecological problems and probably won't treat her if she is pregnant. If she is pregnant, she may consider abortion, but then have trouble finding a clinic willing to treat HIV infected women. More likely, she decides to keep the baby, and face disapproval from some of the health care professionals she must deal with. She fears and has very real concerns for her child's welfare. Even if she can arrange for custody, she wonders how her baby will fare if she dies. Because she may have other children, she may not be available when the HIV/AIDS clinic asks if she can participate in clinical trials, if indeed they ever do. She may seek emotional support, but finds that most of the counseling and support are for gay men and the issues they discuss don't pertain to her. Her family and friends may try to help, but what she really needs is ready access to financial support. However, unless she suffers from a condition recognized by Social Services as AIDS-related, that help may not be forthcoming. By the time all the pieces come together, it may be too late.

These "worst case" scenarios describe the reality of HIV/AIDS for many women in the US. Marking the third annual World AIDS Day, 1 December, 1990, the WHO stated that HIV/AIDS has sweeping social, economic, cultural and political consequences. These conditions are fueling the epidemic, placing women at high risk of acquiring and transmitting the infection. "Therefore, the ultimate solutions to the AIDS pandemic will not be found without acknowledging and addressing these conditions. One of the most critical of these is the status of women." (WHO, 1990, p. 1). Officials at the WHO went on to say that although "AIDS prevention strategies have included a wide range of components...they have yet to address the underlying problem of women's subordination as a factor in the epidemic." (p. 2).

Perception and Acceptance of Risk for HIV/AIDS

Even as HIV educators, policymakers and researchers failed to acknowledge the risks of HIV to women, women were not aware of the risks to themselves. Mays and Cochran (1988) observed that women who feel powerless in sexual, social, economic and political relationships have always lived with risks of some kind. "AIDS is simply one more risk with which to be concerned.... The key to ... women's response to AIDS is their perception of its danger relative to the hierarchy of other risks present in their lives and the existence of resources available to act differently." (p. 951). More immediate concerns, such as economic survival for themselves and their children, often take precedence.

Worth (1990) has observed that many women do not acknowledge risk of infection until a crisis occurs, eg. a partner becomes infected or the prenatal clinic asks for HIV testing. Many women delay because they know they will be forced to re-evaluate their lifestyles, eg. make major changes in economic, sexual and/or drug-associated relationships. Many feel powerless to make these changes on their own. Carpenter *et al.* (1991) found a significant trend towards earlier testing and diagnosis in women in recent years, resulting in higher CD4 counts at the time of presentation. The trend was most obvious among IVDAs who were required to submit to testing as a condition of incarceration or entry into drug treatment programs. The trend was less striking in women at risk for heterosexual transmission, where the incidence of HIV is increasing most rapidly. The most common reason women gave for requesting the HIV test was self-perception of risk. The perception of HIV risk, however, must be balanced against the needs of children, the potential loss of companionship and economic support and the complexity and inflexibility of social systems that provide supplemental help.

Risk Reduction and the Status of Women

Sexual relationships
A woman's ability to reduce her risks for HIV/AIDS is partially a function of how much power she holds in relationships that place her at risk. Sexual relationships may be the most difficult to negotiate. People do not always consider the consequences of risk-taking behaviors when in love (*Newsweek*, 1991, December 9, p. 52), or when sex serves to bolster self-esteem (Worth, 1990) or functions as a commodity (eg. in exchange for drugs [Booth *et al.*, 1991]).

In love relationships, mutual trust is essential. However, the dominant partner in a heterosexual relationship – usually the man – often dictates the terms of that trust. In these situations, all women, poor or middle-class, minority or white, are at risk. Women are often the first to acquiesce to preserve relationships. Sharon T., a white, middle-class attorney, reported to *Newsweek* (1991, December 9) that she felt it was more important to make peace with her husband than insist he wear condoms after she questioned his fidelity. If she trusted him, he argued, she would not demand he wear condoms. "Safe sex is an option [says Sharon], but at some point you have to draw the line and leave it in the hands of providence." (p. 54)

When Janice J., an articulate HIV infected African-American woman, found out her husband had contracted AIDS as a result of intravenous drug abuse, she continued having unprotected sex with him to comfort him during his illness (Brown, 1991). "He wouldn't use a condom; he was suffering and wounded, ... I'm his wife; whatever comes I'm supposed to take it." (p. 86). After nearly two years of psychotherapy, Janice now understands that her low self-esteem had placed her at high risk of HIV infection.

Notwithstanding self-esteem or power issues, a woman can engage unwittingly in 'high risk' sex because she is unaware of her partner's infidelity or bisexuality. We have found this to be the most usual scenario in our research with military women (Brown and Rundell, 1990; in press).

Behavioral change strategies focus on four straightforward issues to prevent heterosexual transmission: (1) partner selection; (2) numbers of partners; (3) mode of sexual expression; and (4) condom use (Stein, 1990). For many women, these issues are problematic. Each implies that women have real choices in sexual relationships. Rarely are the social and psychological aspects considered in the educational design (WHO, 1991). For example, consistent and proper condom use is still considered an important protective behavior for controlling the spread of HIV. On 31 January, 1992, a Food and Drug Administration advisory panel approved a woman's condom ("Reality") to give women more control in sexual decision-making (Gladwell, 1992). Although quite promising, it is expensive ($2.25 per condom) and may require more motivation and skill to use than traditional condoms.

However, women do not wear traditional condoms and, therefore, have no direct control over this behavior. They must rely on men to *accept* the suggestion to wear condoms. Condom acceptability is highly dependent on social, cultural, economic, political and sexual conditions (Worth, 1989). Condom use is not normative in many cultures (WHO, 1991) and even when it is, consistency is dependent on specific situations. When sex is exchanged for drugs or money, a woman's leverage is the value placed on her services and she is often given more money for sex *without* condoms. In relationships, a woman's leverage is her perception of power in sexual decision-making (Stein, 1990).

We have found that women, attempting to engage in behavioral change strategies, often find it very difficult to convince their partners to use condoms. Most often, they use the other three strategies, that is, change partners, have less sex, or limit themselves to one partner (Worth, 1990). Unless interventions are targeted to the man or couple, traditional condom use as a prevention strategy will fall far short of the mark.

For minority women, the situation is further complicated by a high rate of bisexual behavior in their partners (Chu *et al.*, 1992). Chu *et al.* found that the 1989 rate for AIDS in women resulting from sex with a bisexual man was 5 and 3 times higher among African-American and Latina women, respectively, than among white women. Many men do not acknowledge or disclose their bisexuality or same-sex behaviors (Johnson *et al.*, 1990) and would rather admit drug use. Further, Latino men often do not consider themselves bisexual if they are the dominant partners in their homosexual encounters (Mitchell and Heagarty, 1991). There is also evidence that bisexual minority group men engage in certain behaviors more frequently than white men (ie. more receptive anal intercourse [Peterson and Marin, 1988]), further compounding the risks to a woman if the man is HIV infected. Finally, Beral *et al.* (1990) found that the incidence of Kaposki's sarcoma was 4 times higher in women with heterosexually acquired HIV whose partners were bisexual than for women with other sexual partners.

Bringing men and women together to "share the challenge" in combatting heterosexual transmission was the theme of the fourth annual World AIDS Day, 1

December, 1991 (WHO, 1991, p. 1). The WHO suggests several strategies to reduce the inequality between the sexes and increase the use of safer sex behaviors, among them: debunking 'male image' problems regarding condom use, targetting and empowering men (not just women) in family planning programs, balancing sex and sexuality in education and intensive advertising and distribution of condoms in schools and red light districts.

Open, sensitive communication (between partners, parents and children) is an important key to equalizing the balance of power. Generations of sexual repression make this difficult to achieve in the short-run. Young men and women fear being labelled promiscuous and risk rejection for bringing up the subject of safer sex behaviors with potential partners. They avoid the real issues or simply do not perceive themselves to be at risk. Lying about one's sexual history is common. Marks, Richardson and Maldonado (1991) found 52 percent of HIV positive men did not disclose their serostatus to their sexual partners.

In some communities, particularly Latino, cultural barriers to discussing sex and using condoms are strong (Marin *et al.*, 1988; Mays and Cochran, 1988). Latina women (but not men) are expected to enter relationships virginal in body and mind and it has been estimated that at least 25 percent of Latino men oppose the use of condoms (Poma, 1987). Marin *et al.* (1988) reported that the Latino men in their study insisted that penetrative sex was necessary, suggesting that abstinence or alternative sexual behaviors would not be acceptable as preventive strategies. This partially explains why Carpenter *et al.* (1991) found 67 percent of Latina HIV seropositive women had been infected heterosexually, versus 29 percent and 38 percent for white and African-American women, respectively.

In the age of HIV/AIDS, sexual silence can be deadly. Men and women must insist on self-protection; this means knowing the serostatus of their partners and prospective partners and emphasizing the need for periodic HIV testing of themselves and their partners. The WHO (1991) suggests initially targetting educational strategies at single-sex groups to make it easier to break down cultural taboos. Group participants can discuss options and build skills for use in real situations. Educational interventions developed must be tailored to the intended audience.

Schools across the US reported increases in requests by students for HIV testing following Magic Johnson's announcement of his seroconversion. Unfortunately, most of the reported changes were short-term or restricted to individuals who already perceived themselves to be at risk. Cleary *et al.* (1991) found that the strongest predictors of continued risky behaviors after a positive test were engaging in risky behaviors just prior to the test. Equally discouraging, Carpenter *et al.* (1991) found that heterosexuals continue to be the least likely individuals to view themselves as at risk. Undoubtedly, we need to learn more about the reasons why people engage in risky behaviors in order to develop more effective interventions.

Childbearing: Difficult choices

In 1985, the CDC recommended that HIV infected women forgo childbearing until more was known about the risks of perinatal transmission. Early retrospective studies of women with AIDS found a wide range of estimates for the rate of perinatal transmission (0–65 percent) (Andiman and Modlin, 1991). More recent prospective studies of asymptomatic infected women found 13–30 percent of children infected (eg.

European Collaborative Study, 1991). Thirty percent is the currently accepted estimate in the US and in Europe (Oxtoby, 1990).

Because of the long latency period for the development of AIDS, the CDC has collaborated with state and local health departments to collect newborn blood samples from routine metabolic studies in order to monitor trends in HIV seroprevalence (CDC, 1990). Gwinn *et al.* (1991) estimated that 1800 infants were infected perinatally in one year (1990), exceeding the total of 1628 children with AIDS reported to the CDC from 1981 through 1989 (Oxtoby, 1990).

The estimates of maternal-fetal transmission rates have improved but the prognosis for children with AIDS has not. Pediatric AIDS is the ninth leading cause of death in children 1–4 years of age in the US (Novello *et al.*, 1989). Uninfected children also face an uncertain future. The same conditions that placed the family at risk for HIV may still persist. Children are being neglected by ill, drug abusing and dying parents and when orphaned, are left at the mercy of the courts and underfunded social services systems.

Nonetheless, HIV infected women are having babies. "They are doing so even when they know they are infected, even when they have been counseled about the risks of perinatal transmission, even when they already have a child with HIV infection or AIDS and even when that child has died." (Levin and Dubler, 1990, p. 321). In a 4-year prospective study of middle-class seropositive women, one-third had become pregnant at least once since becoming infected (Brown and Rundell, in press).

For women with few options, reproductive freedom is crucial. For many, having children is integral to their biological and social lives, often tied to hopes and dreams that cannot be realized in other ways (Pivnick *et al.*, 1991). The positive cultural value attached to childbearing among African Americans and Latinos may partially explain the decisions to conceive in these populations even with the threat of spreading HIV (Mitchell and Heagarty, 1991). Moreover, public health efforts to prevent pregnancy are viewed by some minorities "as part of a plan for genocide." (Levine and Dubler, 1990, p. 333).

In an attempt to refute the view that HIV infected women who bear children are "immoral", Levine and Dubler (p. 322) described the "values, norms, and practices encompassing women's sexual and reproductive lives – a moral universe – and the economic, cultural, and social reality from which it is derived." The authors, like many others, fully support (informed) voluntary HIV testing and counseling programs *as a gateway to services for women*. However, they are concerned that such programs also provide an expedient way to force women to prevent or abort a pregnancy. For example, although it is illegal to coerce HIV infected pregnant women into sterilization at delivery, in practice such coercion has been reported. At present, we feel there is no easy solution to the very real societal concerns of caring for sick children of dead mothers. Because most children at risk from HIV/AIDS in the US are born to poor, drug abusing, African-American or Latina women, any discussion of families at risk cannot be separated from this context.

The interrelationships of poverty, drug abuse, and ethnicity

Poverty is an underlying social determinant complicating reproductive decision-making. Poverty limits access to educational and economic opportunities that reward delayed childbearing (Levine and Dubler, 1990). Early onset of sexual activity and limited knowledge of contraception lead to early and repeated pregnancies.

Poverty and its consequences force women to relinquish children to relatives or child welfare agencies. Losing custody heightens a sense of loss in infected women who feel they may not live long enough to see a child raised to adulthood. This, in turn, affects these women's decisions to try to replace the lost children. Pivnick *et al.* (1991) found HIV infected drug abusing women more likely to conceive if they had never lived with any of their existing children throughout the children's lives. They found this to be the only major difference between HIV positive women who conceived and those who did not. It is also unlikely that the drug abusing mother will be able to keep her child after birth. Carpenter *et al.* (1991) found only 25 percent of children of infected IVDAs lived with their mothers compared with 92 percent of children of mothers infected heterosexually.

Poor women at risk for HIV/AIDS, especially those with children, often depend on high-risk partners and/or the social services and Medicaid systems for survival (Mitchell and Heagarty, 1991). The systems they must confront are so complex that only the most socially organized and well-represented individuals can successfully negotiate them. Unfortunately, many poor families are very socially disorganized and isolated. They depend on social services for economic and medical support, which limits their choices. At the same time, the services provided must meet their needs. Dynamic education and outreach from professional and grass roots organizations (eg. The Body Positive, The Minority Task Force on AIDS, New York; Blacks Educating Blacks About Sexual Health Issues, Philadelphia), and newsletters (eg. *The Positive Woman*, Washington, DC), have helped HIV infected women learn about the disease, become active participants in their health care and protect themselves and their families. Moving from 'knowledgeable' to 'active' participant is by no means an easy task. Limited economic and personal freedom impedes a smooth transition to preventive behaviors. Complicating matters are racial conditions that spawned and perpetuate longstanding minority distrust of public health authorities (Thomas and Quinn, 1991).

Thomas and Quinn, in their review of the Tuskegee Syphilis Study, in which thousands of syphilis-infected African-American men went untreated until death, observed that the current social conditions and the strategies presently used to recruit participants into HIV/AIDS risk reduction and clinical trials programs are similar to the conditions and strategies that prevailed during the 40-year (1932–1972) course of the Tuskegee study p. 1500–1501. It is no wonder, then, that HIV/AIDS prevention activities have rekindled fears of genocide and are viewed with suspicion by many African Americans.

To reestablish credibility, Thomas and Quinn recommend public health authorities openly discuss the fears of genocide and emphasize disease prevention and treatment. Consistent financial and technical support should be given to community-based organizations which have earned minority trust. Moreover, to ensure successful recruitment, retention and client adherence in clinical and behavioral intervention trials, protocols should be conducted at convenient settings that provide social and outreach services, ancillary support (eg. meals, child care, transportation) and use specialized educational materials (El-Sadr and Capps, 1992). The best approach to achieving favorable results is to provide adequate funding for HIV education and treatment in concert with encouraging testing, condom use and abstinence and providing information about abortion.

When opportunities are constrained by poverty, illicit drug use may become an appealing escape. Profits made from the drug culture lessen the likelihood that one will seek alternatives. Trading sex for drugs is common barter. In one study, female IVDAs cited 'customers' as their most frequent sexual partners (Booth *et al.*, 1991). When drug abuse is the main social activity, unprotected sex is normative, placing women at high risk for HIV, other STDs and pregnancy.

Intravenous drug abuse is one of the primary risky behaviors that place US women at risk for HIV/AIDS according to a number of recent studies (eg. Des Jarlais *et al.*, 1990). Once a woman reports drug abuse, she is labelled an IVDA. However, it should be noted that these studies do not show that HIV infected female IVDAs became infected as a direct result of their drug use. IVDAs do not stop having sex (risky or otherwise) while taking drugs.

Drug use behaviors may be the most difficult to stop and IVDAs may be the most difficult to educate. For the drug-addicted woman, motivation to change may require a "change in perceived self-efficacy, self-esteem, perceived peer group norms, or beliefs about the controllability of the future." (Mays and Cochran, 1988, p. 952) Further, the ability to use safer sex or low risk drug use behaviors involves overcoming feelings of "powerlessness, sociocultural pressures associated with poverty, or emotional needs for intimacy." (p. 952). These are formidable barriers, but the threat of HIV is beginning to impact upon this discouraging picture.

Mays and Cochran (1988) observed that HIV/AIDS prevention efforts are most successful when offered within the context of the drug culture. Needle exchange programs, and intensive education on cleaning 'works' (injection equipment) and avoiding 'shooting galleries' (needle sharing), are examples of programs that forgo moralism in favor of reality. Similar programs implemented in both Europe and Australia have been shown to be successful (Anderson, 1991). However, Des Jarlais and his colleagues (1990) noted that although the rates of new infections have slowed as a result, they are still rising much faster than among homosexual/bisexual men.

These programs are not without controversy. In recounting the history of the New York City Needle Exchange Program (1985–1991), Anderson (1991) described what can occur when political concerns dictate public health services. The officially sanctioned program[a] was dismantled because special interest groups could not agree on the most politically expedient way to continue the program beyond the designation of a clinical trial.

Among the many arguments that doomed the New York program was the perception that drug abusers desperate for a 'fix' would not care about contaminated needles. Further, it was argued that supplying needles would increase drug use. Neither has been found to be the case in Europe (Flanagan *et al.*, 1988).

To many individuals at risk, HIV/AIDS is seen as more threatening than drug abuse. Studies have shown that HIV education does result in lowered injection drug use among students (Brown, 1991) and risky drug use behaviors among addicts (Booth *et al.*, 1991). Additionally, there is evidence to suggest that effective and ongoing treatment of drug abuse reduces the spread of HIV and the risk of AIDS-related mortality (Selwyn, 1991). However, Selwyn pointed out that the number of addicts seeking treatment far exceeds the number of treatment slots available. Inevitably,

---

[a]Underground needle exchange programs still exist in high drug-use areas; these programs appear to reach more addicts than the official program (Des Jarlais and Stepherson, 1991).

predict Des Jarlais and Stepherson (1991), policymakers will see HIV/AIDS as more threatening than political polemics, and arrive at policies that do protect the public's health.

RESEARCH ON WOMEN: A MULTI-FACETED NATIONAL AGENDA

Research and clinical care issues relevant to women and HIV were the focal points of discussion at the *First National Conference on Women and HIV* (NIAID, CDC, 1991). The purpose of the conference was to: (a) increase awareness of the growing problem of women and HIV: (b) facilitate information-sharing about medical, psychosocial and prevention issues specific to HIV infected women; and (c) formulate recommendations for research. Stressing the need for greater physician vigilance and suggesting directions for new research initiatives were major goals.

At the meeting, the CDC attributed the absence of women-specific conditions in the pre-1992 CDC definition of AIDS and related conditions to a lack of adequate data. US Surgeon General Antonia Novello stated that although the infection rate in women will equal that observed in men by the year 2000, women make up only five percent of the subjects used in experimental drug trials (*The Nation's Health*, 1991, January, p. 4). Rosser (1991) has argued that male researchers take a male approach to problems, but espouse the objectivity of science. This, she says, "makes it difficult for them to admit that they actually hold any perspectives that may influence their data, approaches, and theories." (p. 231). Although this view is not new (eg. see Osborn, 1986), the fact that it has continued means that research findings on women lag far behind data on men.

The proposed study areas listed in Table 7.3 summarize the issues discussed in this chapter. Initial steps have been taken. As of 1 December, 1990, study sections in the National Institutes of Health/Alcohol, Drug Abuse and Mental Health Administration that review HIV/AIDS proposals have incorporated explicit policy instructions to investigators and reviewers. Applicants for clinical research grants, cooperative agreements and contracts are required to include women and minorities in study populations so that research findings can be of benefit to all persons at risk for the disease, disorder, or condition under study. If women or minorities are not included or are inadequately represented in clinical research, particularly in proposed population-based studies, a clear, compelling rationale should be provided.

Following the Washington meeting, the National Conference Steering Committee (composed of health care providers, researchers and women with HIV) made a series of recommendations for use in planning a research agenda. Central to the recommendations was the integration of psychosocial, behavioral and biomedical issues (*The Positive Woman*, 1991, June/July). The committee recommended that ongoing projects and new research proposals be carefully reviewed for compliance with the new policy instructions. Information, funding and technical assistance are to be provided to community-based organizations to enhance outreach and research efforts. Priority funding is to be given to researchers who show substantive collaboration with community-based organizations and primary care providers and to programs which train such organizations to develop their own research methodologies.

For their part, the CDC has moved to expand the definition of AIDS to include

TABLE 7.3
Recommendations for Research on Women and HIV Infection
(Adapted with permission from *The Positive Woman*, 1991, June/July).

1. Transmission and HIV prevention studies:
(a) Study the cofactors and coinfections that play a role in HIV transmission, especially in the female genital tract.
(b) Develop barrier methods that women can control.
(c) Expand and improve drug dependency programs that do not impair mother-child relationships.
(d) Develop behavioral interventions that emphasize the male role in primary prevention.
(e) Monitor the seroprevalence and develop training programs that meet the special *and specific* needs of women, sub-groups of women (eg. adolescents, lesbians, disabled, non-English speaking), and minorities.
2. Progression of HIV disease in women via a large-scale cohort study:
(a) Describe the full spectrum of infections, pre-cancerous lesions and malignancies to fully evaluate AIDS case definitions, determine the relationship between HIV and carcinogenesis, and improve standards of medical care.
(b) Determine the relationship of immune function (eg. via CD4 counts, p24 antigenemia) to women-specific conditions and survival rates in women as compared to men.
(c) Using culturally appropriate methods, investigate factors that may affect neuropsychological and neurobiological functioning and immune function.
(d) Study the psychosocial needs of HIV positive women and their traditional and non-traditional family systems.
3. Treatment and research needs:
(a) Determine the safety and efficacy of therapies to control the virus and opportunistic infections in both pregnant and non-pregnant women, including interactions with other substances (eg. methadone, oral contraceptives).
(b) Include gender-specific clinical assessments (eg. pelvic examinations, Pap smears) in the routine evaluation of an HIV infected woman's medical status.
(c) Review clinical trial eligibility (eg. definitions of active drug use, pregnancy) and evaluate recruitment and retention strategies (eg. access to medical care, support services) that may restrict or prevent many women from participation.
(d) Develop inexpensive, accessible therapeutics which can be used by women who must frequently manage multiple responsibilities (eg. family, job) despite declining health.
(e) Study women's perceptions of the clinical trial process and develop culturally-competent and gender unbiased education and informed consent procedures.
(f) Study the determinants of women's health-seeking behavior and the role of social networks in facilitating access to care. Concomitantly, improve outreach and case finding activities with effective counseling in various settings that are fully linked to medical and social services.
(g) Determine the full extent of services needed to improve access, coordination and quality of care.
(h) Evaluate the adequacy of HIV/AIDS training of health care providers to improve sensitivity, develop effective communication, and effectively change biased attitudes towards HIV infected clients.

anyone with a CD4 cell count of $\leqslant 200/mm^3$, effective in April, 1992 (*CDC AIDS Weekly*, 1991, August, p. 2). The new system standardizes clinical monitoring of HIV by immune function rather than by infection. Although most view this as a distinct improvement, physician vigilance regarding the early signs of HIV in asymptomatic women needs to be enhanced. The Social Security Administration recently revamped its AIDs eligibility requirement to include diseases found in women and children (*The Nation's Health*, 1991, December, p. 4).

The American Foundation for AIDS Research has awarded nearly $800,000 during fiscal year 1991–1992 to fund innovative projects with focused educational objectives (*CDC AIDS Weekly*, 1991, August, p. 8). Included are skill-building programs that teach African-American youth and Latina women in New Jersey how to negotiate safer sex behaviors with their partners. Although these studies deal with small populations, they integrate the psychosocial, behavioral and clinical needs of women.

Most importantly, the new research initiatives recognize the need to empower women to challenge their partners and the social and medical systems. The research and medical communities are directed to integrate, not isolate – to study and provide care in the context of real life, not the laboratory. Further, study results are to be disseminated in a timely manner, providing the education and opportunities necessary for women to participate actively in making the choices which will save their lives.

FURTHER READING

Faden, R.R., Geller, G. and Powers, M. (1991). *AIDS, women, and the next generation: Towards a morally acceptable public policy for HIV testing of pregnant women and newborns*. New York: Oxford University Press.

Wasserheit, J.N., Aral, S.O. and Holmes, K.K. (Eds.). (1991). *Research issues in human behavior and sexually transmitted diseases in the AIDS era*. Washington, DC: American Society for Microbiology.

8

WOMEN, FOOD AND BODY IMAGE

VIVIEN J. LEWIS

Royal Shrewsbury Hospital Shelton, Bicton Heath, Shrewsbury SY3 8DN, UK

ALAN J. BLAIR

19 Hartfield Close, Hasland, Chesterfield, Derbyshire S41 0NU, UK

In the sixteenth century, women with waists measuring more than 13 inches were barred from the court of Catherine de'Medici. Indeed, throughout history women have been given detailed prescriptions about what their appearance and physical dimension should be in order to achieve social acceptability. Like the lines and contours of a modern car, female lines, contours and curves, or the lack of them, have been marketed as commodities, such that what is socially desirable in one decade is stigmatized in the next. Thus the media images objectifying women, past and present, can illustrate the sociocultural ground upon which the figures of distressed eating and distorted body image stand.

In recent history, women have had uneasy relationships with food and with their bodies, in such a way that mirrors their relationship with the cultures within which they have struggled to find identity. The consequence of this in the present time is a gamut of difficulties associated with food and body image, experienced by females of as young as 8 years and well into old age. These difficulties range along the dimension of body weights from the medically constructed category of 'obesity' to the psychiatrically constructed categories of 'anorexia nervosa' and 'bulimia nervosa', and include the experiences of cyclic dieting, binge-eating, vomitting, laxative and/or diuretic use and other health-risking weight-control strategies.

There have been numerous attempts to categorize and classify variants of distressed eating and body image, largely by the medical profession. However, not surprisingly, there is no clear consensus about which features are sufficient or necessary for the diagnoses of 'anorexia nervosa', 'bulimia', 'normal-weight bulimia', 'bulimia nervosa', 'bulimarexia' and so forth. Indeed, the nomenclature itself is inconsistent between, for example, DSM-III R and the International Classification of Disorders and there is a substantial lobby currently, particularly amongst those who have survived the experience of these disorders and the psychiatric treatment there of, that is arguing cogently for the removal of any 'eating disorder' from the diagnostic criteria for 'mental illnesses'.

The feature which appears to be most fundamental to all forms of eating distress, although it is most often ascribed to what is called 'anorexia nervosa', is the pursuit of thinness. Women rarely consciously aspire to being fat in modern Western society. However, those women that are significantly overweight are likely to be subject to the psychological distresses associated with the experience of 'difference' and 'stigmatisation'. They may experience a sense of failure in their ability to conform adequately and engage successfully in self-denial and, paradoxically, may at times comfort overwhelming feelings of guilt by emotional over-eating, thus compounding the experience of failure. The paradox is that those who *succeed* in the pursuit of ultimate and extreme thinness, those individuals who achieve emaciation, may feel exactly the same guilt and failure – thin may never feel thin enough, and the merest morsel may be experienced as over-eating.

This chapter will aim to set the context within which women's distress and disorder about food and body image occurs. A framework for food and body-shape-related behaviour popularly known as 'dieting' will be presented, drawn from social and experimental psychological research. These contexts will then form the background upon which the experience of severe eating distress is drawn. Finally, the chapter will propose approaches for education and enabling intervention which aim to empower women to determine their own balance for food, body and health.

THE HISTORICAL CONTEXT

Many women who perceive themselves as overweight (whether or not they actually are) may wistfully declare that they should have been born a few centuries ago when 'Rubenesque' figures were viewed as the aesthetic ideal. If they *had* been born then, they would also have been subject to other aspects of the experience of womanhood in the seventeenth century. Most notable amongst these was the social construction, reinforced in law, that women were men's property. One consequence of this property relation was that women were viewed as objects and status symbols. Thus the ideal of a rounded and well-fed figure for a woman then (when food was less plentiful), perhaps like a BMW at the present time in Western cultures, functioned as a representation of her husband or father's wealth and status. Artists such as Rubens and Rembrandt portrayed women whose body weights would have been in the region of around 12 or 13 stones if their heights are extrapolated to about 5 foot 4 or 5 inches, body weights which would currently be considered markedly overweight. These aesthetic ideals for women's body shapes were maintained largely until well into the nineteenth century.

By the nineteenth century, however, there began to be a different expression of the dissatisfaction with the ways in which women's roles and potential contributions to society were being restricted. Indeed, in a recent biography of Emily Brontë who died in 1848, the author Katherine Frank argued that Emily Brontë was anorexic and that her condition was the only rebellion she could make against her powerlessness as the daughter of a clergyman in an isolated Yorkshire village, with poor marriage prospects and an almost inevitable fate as a governess (Frank, 1990).

At the present time, there is a debate as to whether what is known as 'anorexia nervosa' today may have been more prevalent historically than has been documented, although construed differently. Alternatively, others contend that 'anorexia nervosa' as described by physicians in the late nineteenth century was not the same as the disorder known by that name today. One perspective is to view the core motivations underlying these disorders as equivalent. Clearly the Romans being sick in their vomitariums during feasts two thousand years ago was an experience markedly different from what is known as 'bulimia nervosa' now, and the spiritual fasting undertaken by some young females from the fourteenth century onwards may differ significantly from what is now known as "anorexia nervosa". Nevertheless, certainly by the nineteenth century, women appeared to be becoming far more aware of the inequalities and contradictions of their experiences both within their families and also within the wider society, to an extent which created a pattern of internal conflicts closely mirroring those experienced by many women today.

Testament to this can be found in the fascinating writings of one of the most famous women of the nineteenth century, Florence Nightingale. In a passage from "Cassandra" written in 1852, Florence Nightingale wrote:

"Why have women passion, intellect, moral activity – these three – and a place in society where no one of the three can be exercised? ... Women often long to enter some man's profession where they would find direction, competition (or rather the opportunity of measuring the intellect with others) and, above all, time. ... A woman dedicates herself to the vocation of her husband; she fills up and performs the subordinate parts in it. But if she has any destiny, any vocation of her own, she must renounce it, in nine cases out of ten." (pp. 246–249).

Florence Nightingale also makes an interesting observation on women in relation to food:

"If she has a knife and fork in her hand for three hours of the day, she cannot have a pencil or brush. Dinner is the great sacred ceremony of this day, the great sacrament. To be absent from dinner is equivalent to being ill. Nothing else will excuse us from it. Bodily incapacity is the only apology valid." (p. 245).

Less than 20 years later, William Withey Gull in Britain and E.C. Lasegue in France, both physicians, identified what is now known as 'anorexia nervosa' (Gull, 1874; Lasegue, 1873). At that time, the context within which the discovery of this 'disorder' was set, was one of a medical model which linked the possession of a uterus to a variety of forms of biologically based insanity. In 1871, G. Fielding Blandford of the Psychiatric Section of the British Medical Association wrote:

"Women become insane during pregnancy, after parturition, during lactation; at the age when the catamenia (menses) first appear and when they disappear (the menopause). The sympathetic connection between the brain and the uterus is plainly seen by the most casual observer." (p. 71).

This argument, which was often used to restrict women's access to higher education, was based on the belief that too much education might damage a woman's uterus and hence impair the major life task of bearing and nurturing children. Identifying 'anorexia nervosa' as published in 1874, Gull stated:

"The want of appetite is, I believe, due to a morbid mental state. I have not observed in these cases any gastric disorder to which the want of appetite could be referred. I believe, therefore, that its origin is central and not peripheral. That mental states may destroy appetite is notorious, and it will be admitted that young women at the ages named are specially obnoxious to mental perversity." (p. 25).

Referring to the treatment of these "mentally perverse" young women, Gull stated:

"The treatment required is obviously that which is fitted for persons of unsound mind. The patients should be fed at regular intervals, and surrounded by persons who would have moral control over them; relations and friends being generally the worst attendants." (p. 26).

Interestingly, more than 100 years later, in many places the treatment is very little changed from that originally propounded by Gull.

The advent of the twentieth century brought many changes for both men and women in Western societies. In 1906 the movement for women's suffrage became active in Britain, although women in Britain were not finally enfranchised until after the First World War. The esthetic ideal for women's body shapes continued to change, perhaps best exemplified by the well-known quotation from Wallis Simpson, the Duchess of Windsor, who said that a woman could never be "too rich or too thin". Women had the vote and were gradually beginning to receive higher education on a larger scale in the years prior to the Second World War.

Within Britain during the course of the Second World War, the working male population gradually diminished as men were involved in active combat. This led to a shortage of workers essential for wartime production and consequently to the recruitment of women for occupations previously undertaken predominantly by men. This meant that women were taken out of the domestic environment and placed in positions of responsibility and decision-making which ranged beyond the immediate family. However in the post-War period, when men returning from combat re-entered the labour force, women (who had formed a "reserve army of labor") were pressurized to give up their positions of paid employment and relative independence. Indeed, an overt campaign was organized, which encouraged women to return to the 'kitchens', in other words, the site of their traditional role in food preparation and nurturing. This campaign re-emphasized women's household roles, including mothering and the purchase, preparation and provision of food. Even more striking, within the arena of the family, women's relationship with food came to symbolize a vehicle for the transmission of emotional nurturance and love (Orbach, 1986).

Since the Second World War, the documented incidence of difficulties associated with food and body image has increased dramatically. Conceivably part of the explanation for this lies in the changes that women have experienced both within the family and within the wider social context. While women began to receive better education, albeit often only to be used until the woman became attached to a man and took on the traditional domestic duties, the aesthetically idealized body shape was gradually decreasing. Eventually a new role model began to prevail for the young female, or at least for the young white Western middle-class female. This role model was a woman who was educated and engaged in paid employment until such point as she stopped to take on the tasks of housewife and mother. In the 1960s, physical role models became increasingly thin, exemplified by a young fashion model called Twiggy. Among the dominant messages communicated to white middle class women were: "Be thin, but feed others", "Be educated, but sacrifice your training in order to nurture others", or alternatively, "Be both, be mother and career person, be superwoman!"

In order to help women achieve the socially constructed and prescribed body shape, over recent years diet and slimming products and magazines have proliferated. Many magazines are devoted exclusively to the pursuit of the ideal body shape. Furthermore, general magazines for women inevitably include slimming sections, with the latest gimmick for losing those surplus pounds. With no apparent sense of irony, some of them have a slimming diet on one page, cake recipes and advertisements for chocolates on others, closely followed by a section on eating disorders on another. Similarly health and fitness magazines often have a back section devoted to what the reader should do if she has gone too far with her quest for the optimum physique.

The media frequently presents confusing messages: chocolate is bad for you, chocolate can be good for you; sugar is bad, sugar is a natural part of our diet. Also, there has been conflicting information published over recent years about white and brown bread, cholesterol, fibre, saturated fats and so forth. A dieting book from the 1960s, "The Complete Woman Book of Successful Slimming" perhaps exemplifies this (Woman Magazine publications, 1966). Contained in it as a recommendation for weight loss were foods which are largely discouraged in the 1990s, such as eggs and bacon for a dieting breakfast and for 'average speed weight loss' one could eat in 'any quantity' such things as butter, cream, dripping, duck and hazelnuts. In contradiction, in a virtual prescription for what is known as 'anorexia nervosa', this dieting book also proposes the "Start-Right Diet", where the total energy intake for 1 day would be 3 crispreads and butter, 1 cup of fresh orange juice, 1 pint of milk (in tea/coffee if preferred), 1 Marmite or similar drink, and 1 portion of clear soup (with bouillon cube or consomme). In this regard it is noteworthy that it is commonly the case that women (and not men) express a wish to weigh significantly less not only than that which they themselves perceive would be healthier, but also significantly less than that which they perceive would be most attractive for themselves (Lewis and Booth, 1986).

So the context today, within which 'eating disorders' are situated, is one in which there is much conflict and contradiction. Society is still strongly gender-stratified and it might be argued that women have been hoist on their own petards. Striving for equal opportunities with men, some women feel guilty if they work and choose not to have a family, some feel guilty if they raise a family and do not contribute overtly to the family income, some try to do both and feel guilty because they become afraid they are doing neither well enough. For the adolescent and young adult female entering this state of apparent role conflict, retreat into the arena of food consumption, one of the few opportunities for experiencing control, may appear to be an attractive solution. Indeed dietary chaos can stand as a metaphor for the individual's sociopsychological distress.

DIETING

The arguments above serve as an attempt to set the general historical and social context for what has been described as an 'epidemic' of difficulties associated with food and body image, where well in excess of 50 percent of the female population in Britain experience such problems to some extent, if only through frequent, often unsuccessful, active attempts at weight control and through body dissatisfaction. As has been demonstrated, one of the strongest and most common current concerns about health among women in Western cultures is to eat and drink in a way that seeks to attain or maintain a slim body shape. Such uses of foods and drinks are popularly known as 'dieting'. Whether slimming or weight loss is desired because of health considerations, socio-cultural ideals or other factors, it provides one of the most powerful motivations for dietary change in people not actually suffering from any specific health disorder. A 'healthy weight' is taken to be that range of body weight relative to height for which there is no evidence of significant risk to mortality or morbidity.

An effective conception of dieting has to work within the facts of physics: except for transient water losses, weight loss requires a period of negative energy balance and the maintenance of that loss requires the avoidance subsequently of any running-average positive energy balance. For anybody, an appropriate level of exercise is worth attaining and maintaining. However, the greatest scope for achieving negative energy balance is a reduction in energy intake relative to that individual's own intake when gaining weight or maintaining overweight. In addition, there may be changes in lifestyle that are necessary over and above whatever can be done about energy expenditure. In what is known as 'anorexia nervosa', of course, these are taken to the extreme.

The thermodynamics of dieting therefore requires the learning of dietary habits and preferences likely to result in lower energy intake together with the monitoring of their impact on body weight over time in the particular individual. 'Success' is eating sufficiently less to move towards a healthy weight, however slowly. Failure is either never eating that much less, stopping eating that much less too soon, eating that much less for too long, or alternating eating much less with eating much more.

The physics of dieting is straightforward, but the sociology, psychology and physiology of dieting and dietary behavior generally are far more complex. There are many myths unscrupulously or unintentionally promoted about eating less without eating less, but nutritional psychology is highly individual. Maintenance of desirable body weight in the end depends entirely on the individual agent. There are many ways for an individual to reduce intake and maintain that reduction for as long as is necessary given his or her metabolism and given some level of physical activity. The appropriate behavior for an individual in his or her circumstances is a psychological matter, provided that dietary practices are changed in a direction that is realistically liable to reduce energy intake and is evaluated against the weighing scales.

Intentional dieting has a rationale comprised of various evaluative beliefs about the practicality and efficacy of particular sorts of behavior. Various theoretical models have been developed which provide descriptions of the relationships among beliefs, reasons, attitudes and reported behavior, and which, in some cases attempt to predict observed behavior. But beliefs and values about body shape and weight cannot directly influence eating and other related behavior or connect up with food beliefs and values, without some intervening process. Such reasoning is likely to involve evaluations of the importance of various beliefs which may contribute to the intentions to perform various acts.

Two approaches to structuring attitude analysis are well known, the Behavioural Intentions Model (Fishbein and Ajzen, 1975; Sejwacz *et al.*, 1980) and the Health Belief Model (Becker *et al.*, 1977). The predictive power of these approaches depends on the individual's freedom of action or at least on the individual's ability in their expressed reasoning to allow for constraints on choice (such as lack of opportunity or money) and counter-influences (such as emotional factors or tempting foods). When the questioning is specific to types of behavior in common situations where there truly is full discretion, such attitudes may be moderately predictive of behavior. In dieting, over-dieting, or intermittent dieting, then, these attitudinal structures may underpin the rational or quasi-rational cognitions contributing to the maintenance of the situation.

However, attempting to lose, maintain or gain weight is rarely a purely rational, directly verbalisable matter. For example, a substantial proportion of obese and normal-weight people are afflicted with a habit of emotional overeating, without it necessarily falling into the category of what is called an 'eating disorder'. This emotional overeating is especially likely to occur when emotions are experienced as 'diffuse' and uncontrollable, and this pattern of eating may be characterized as a learned strategy for coping with emotions which are unpleasant to the individual. Elsewhere in this text Graham and Bancroft suggest that the ingestion of sugars has an anti-depressant effect.

Some overweight people experience a higher incidence of emotional eating, particularly in response to anxiety, loneliness or depression (Slochower and Kaplan, 1980). Furthermore, emotional eating interferes with attempts to lose weight and volitional breakdowns occurring among those attempting body weight control or reduction most often happen in response to mood pressure due to strong emotional stress. Similarly, after successful dieting, those who regain body weight report eating in response to various states of emotional arousal. For a serious dieter, this mechanism might sometimes lead to a vicious spiral of overeating in response to guilt or worry at some real or imaginary breach of the diet and hence an anxiety-mediated breakdown of dietary restraint. dietary restraint.

Another psychological theory of difficulties in dietary weight control, proposed by Schachter and his colleagues (eg. Schachter and Rodin, 1974), is that some individuals have a personality trait of high involuntary responsiveness to salient external stimuli of all types. Schachter (1971) assumed that 'externality' was associated with obesity per se. However, this trait has proved not to relate to physical overweight specifically but rather to psychological problems in weight control. These include, for example, weight gain on moving into an environment with more attractive dietary choices and a poor ability to learn to react to food stimuli according to their satiating effects on the body (Rodin, 1981).

Some years ago a proposition was made by Nisbett (1972) that any individual, whether normal-weight or obese, might eat in order to bring their weight into line with some biologically determined 'set point'. Individual differences in 'set point' would then account for individual differences in eating behavior and body weight. So, individuals could differ with respect to the extent to which their current weight corresponded to their biologically determined 'set point' weight. If an individual was underweight with respect to his or her 'set point' weight (whether or not they were underweight per se), then that individual would be food-deprived and effectively permanently hungry.

However, there is no actual evidence to support the existence of a physiological comparison mechanism acting in accordance with the deviation of some real bodily characteristic from a 'preferred' value of that characteristic. Nevertheless, a 'settling point' rather than 'set point' might be established if social, psychological and physiological factors are in equilibrium and the idea of a 'set point' has given way more recently to the concept of a regulatory 'boundary' (Polivy and Herman, 1985).

Based on Schachter and Nisbett's propositions, Herman and his co-workers claimed that over-responsiveness was not an inherent personality characteristic, but rather the arousal or general responsiveness resulting from self-deprivation of food (Herman and Polivy, 1980). If this was the case then emotional responsiveness should result from successful dieting and weight loss, but the evidence for this is not consistent.

Herman and his co-workers had showed that some people tended to take a large snack after they had eaten some food in what purported to be a taste test. Indeed, the more these people had taken during 'tasting', the more they ate in the immediately subsequent snack. This 'counterregulatory' response was to the perceived energy eaten, not to the actual energy, and the people showing this response scored highly in a questionnaire devised by Herman (1978). This Dietary Restraint Questionnaire was composed to tap current spasmodic attempts at self-restraint, which the researchers considered to be a syndrome involving a tangle of worry and binges or splurges, with resultant variations in body weight. The dieters were not necessarily obese, some were at medically normal weight. This weight is defined to be a Body Mass Index (ie. weight/height^2) within the range 20 to 24.9. It was found, however, that the low scorers on the Questionnaire did not show "breakdown of restraint" in the experimental test and that they ate less at the snack the more they thought they had eaten previously.

There is evidence that those who score highly on the Dietary Restraint Questionnaire do counterregulate in consequence of such factors as alcohol, depression, observation and modelling (Herman *et al.*, 1979). However, the pattern of scores on this Questionnaire does not differentiate between obese and normal weight individuals. Although it is a valid predictor of experimental results in student populations, the items on the Dietary Restraint Questionnaire are extremely diverse. Indeed, they reflect quite different processes in the general population, especially in representative dieters. Several research studies have shown that responses to the questions on weight variation intercorrelate better amongst themselves than they do with most of the other questions, which tend to form at least one other dimension (Ruderman, 1986). Also clinically obese people may have a more complex factor structure than people in the normal weight range (Lowe, 1984).

Some items on the Dietary Restraint Questionnaire concern the emotionality of dieting, while others concern particular behavior patterns and others the frequency of or attention to dieting in general terms. These different items do not represent a single variable, but rather the 'dietary restraint' construct itself breaks down empirically into various practices, their impact on weight and various intentions, attitudes and emotional experiences.

Dieting is clearly a multidimensional phenomenon and dieting behavior involves the adoption of a repertoire of procedures believed by the individual to facilitate the loss of body weight. The complex psychobiosocial system of dieting comprises a network of the relationships between cognitive, physiological and behavioral processes involved in dieting within a gender-related social and historical context.

Dieting behaviors can range over all food choices, but are rationally and emotionally linked in with loss of (and failure to lose) supposedly excess weight. Belief in one's own ability to carry out a dieting procedure as well as a health-related belief of personal susceptibility to overweight appear to be crucial factors in predicting intentions to act

(Bandura, 1977). Further research is needed in order to elucidate those factors which are involved in an individual's perception of the relevance to him or her of a particular risk. More needs to be known about the role of self-confidence and confidence in the ability to carry out particular behaviors. Therapy and education are likely to be far more successful if such beliefs can be enhanced. For example, personal effectiveness training may go some way to promoting increased confidence and be a necessary component of therapy for body weight control (whether in terms of loss, gain or maintenance).

Dietary behaviors, therefore, are associated with food-specific and other reasoning that includes elements of the Health Belief Model, of the self-efficacy that is so important in behavior changes and of the reasons for action assessed by the Behavioral-Intentions model. The Inventories for 'Dietary Restraint' and 'External Responsiveness', however, do not represent unitary styles of life or personality traits. Trait approaches, therefore, cannot fully account for the complex nature of behavior such as dieting. Indeed, network structure is essential for the measurement of the relative influences of individuals' expressed reasoning and emotions (as well as sensory preferences) on their actual selection of particular foods for consumption.

DISTRESS

As evidenced from a variety of epidemiological studies, adolescence appears to be a time of increased vulnerability to developing an eating disorder. The processes involved in the aetiology of eating disorders are far from clear, however.

The occurrence of eating disorders has been associated with a multitude of factors including dysfunctional family dynamics, the experience of sexual abuse, affective disorder, the possession of various personality characteristics such as perfectionistic striving, low self-esteem, attachment and separation difficulties, and maladaptive early childhood eating behavior. In addition, there is weak putative evidence for a genetic component in the development of what are known as the 'eating disorders'.

Separate from the above, there is also a copious literature on the sociocultural aspects of the development of eating disorders. One facet of this is the increasingly documented "culture of slenderness" (Leon, 1980; Wooley and Wooley, 1984). Certainly, adolescent females, in particular, are subject to powerful social messages with regard to body shape, as previously discussed. This is reflected in the large proportion who reveal a desire to lose weight. For example, one study using a British sample reported that this desire was experienced in approximately one-quarter of females aged 11 and 12 (Salmons *et al.*, 1988). That such a proportion increases markedly throughout the teenage years was demonstrated in another study which found that, by 17 years old, 84 percent of US females desired weight loss (Whitaker *et al.*, 1989).

Such concerns can be seen as motivating a high occurrence of attempts actively to control weight. For example, in a survey of over 1000 females in a Chicago suburb, it was found that, by 14 years of age, 52 percent had already engaged in at least one episode of dieting (Johnson *et al.*, 1983). Such findings are particularing concerning given that dieting has been identified as a precursor to eating disordered behavior. Also, it has been reported that females who, early in adolescence, felt most negatively about their body, were more likely to develop eating problems. Perhaps significantly, the incidence of eating disordered behavior is particularly high in adolescent groups who are especially focussed on body weight or shape, such as professional dance students, ballet students, cheerleaders and athletes.

While authors adopting a sociocultural perspective generally acknowledge the powerful role of weight concerns and dieting behavior, some have argued that other sociocultural influences are equally or more important. Crisp (1984), for example, suggested that society's degree of structure and limit setting was also implicated. Crisp postulated that this influence occurred through religious and secular customs and institutions and through society's values and concerns in relation to the adolescent female's developing impulses, her feelings of competence and self-esteem, as well as her family's value systems.

It can also be argued that a narrow focus on social pressures regarding body shape ignores the more pervasive patriarchal discourses which currently ascribe social value to females through their physical appearance. It has been suggested that women's bodies are seen as available to the 'public gaze'. Such a gaze falls not only upon shape but also upon, for example, hair and clothing. Thus, a variety of service industries serve both to reflect and reinforce the cultural message that women should be valued in terms of their appearance. It is not surprising, therefore, that the body can become a site of resistance to this dominant discourse. Indeed, from such a perspective eating disordered behavior has been conceptualized by, for example, Orbach (1986) as reflecting ambivalence about such social pressures, simultaneously symbolizing a rejection and an exaggeration of the idealized female form.

The prevailing discourses are made increasingly dysfunctional for women if we take the perspective that females are subject to a variety of contradictory pressures in modern Western cultures. These conflicting pressures have been described as 'passive-dependent' and 'assertive-dependent' and it has been argued that the period of adolescence is the time at which females first begin to experience these conflicting expectations fully. For Marilyn Lawrence (1984), crises with regard to autonomy and independence are most commonly experienced in adolescence and it is the failure to resolve these crises which leads to the development of eating-disordered behavior.

From the above observations, it is clear that adolescence is often a crucial period in the development of an eating disorder. Such an observation raises the question of whether it is possible to intervene successfully with adolescents with the aim of reducing the risk of developing an eating disorder. In this context, it is noteworthy that among the recent developments in primary prevention is a focus on children and adolescents, particularly within the school setting. If, as has been argued, preventive interventions aimed at school-aged children are an important part of an overall prevention strategy, then schools can be viewed as one of the most potent media through which such a strategy can be enacted. The high-impact environment of school has the double advantage of the institutionalized structure to reach primarily 'healthy' populations coupled with the opportunity to develop programmes for 'at risk' individuals, while potentially minimising the stigmatization that accompanies many mental health interventions. The school, therefore, is a possible site through which the risk of eating disorders in adolescent females may be addressed.

While early preventive interventions are valuable, there continues to be a need for health care professionals to engage in individual or group therapy or education with women who are experiencing distress related to food and body image. While some of these women might be medically defined as having an 'eating disorder', there is also a broader group of women who, although not diagnosed as 'eating disordered', experience low self-esteem and low self-efficacy as a consequence of concern about their eating behavior and physical appearance (Cooper *et al.*, 1984).

EDUCATION AND ENABLEMENT

For both groups, education and therapy need to aim to enable individuals to acquire the appropriate knowledge and skills, which they can incorporate effectively into their own life-styles. The emphasis should be on both increased personalization of programmes of information and skill transfer and also on the importance of the social contexts in which individuals live. Therapists should no longer 'treat' the 'client' for 'obesity' or 'bulimia' or "anorexia nervosa". Instead, individuals should be empowered to determine their own balance of values between appearance and health; individuals should be enabled, where appropriate, to choose sustainable habits of eating and exercise that could contribute substantially to negative energy balance, and to avoid situations which could undermine their intentions to attain a particular body weight. Weight change per se should not be the focus of intervention or education but, rather, self-efficacy in weight control and self-assertion in body image should be encouraged.

Thus, therapeutic approaches might comprise information-giving about the behavior of dieting and also about dietary health-risk factors. Nutritional and dietary education could be included as well as information about exercise, behavioral strategies and practical supports which have been found to be effective in facilitating permanent loss of body weight (Blair *et al.*, 1989).

With regard to the moderation of dieting emotions, in particular emotional overeating and binge-eating, an adaptation of Beck's (1976) cognitive therapeutic approaches could be incorporated. Then, logically building on to these first two components, therapy could include approaches intended to increase personal effectiveness, such as assertion training both with a generic orientation and also with a more specific focus on issues of food and body shape. Finally, but also arising throughout the course of therapy, common reasons for dieting and attitudes to female appearance might be elucidated, with a view to enabling self-assertion against social pressure on women (Lewis and Blair, 1991).

We have utilized such therapeutic procedures with significant and maintained improvements in reported self-esteem, self-efficacy and assertiveness (Lewis *et al.*, 1992). Emotional eating was also reduced, as was variability in dieting practices. This approach does not emphasize weight reduction in overweight and obese individuals (except where there are associated health reasons) and, indeed, in recent work with individuals labelled as suffering from 'anorexia nervosa', (where possible) weight gain is not emphasized. Nevertheless, in these groups of mostly overweight women a significant amount of weight was lost during therapy; this was maintained and their body weights were further reduced at follow-up.

This integrated structure for food and body weight related behavior also informs a therapeutic approach for what are known as the 'eating disorders' and in particular 'bulimia nervosa' and 'anorexia nervosa'. Such an approach, in some respects, is not that different from cognitive-behavioral techniques (eg. Cooper and Fairburn, 1984) and Orbach's (1985) feminist model.

The starting point is a very simple contract, involving an agreement to see the individual on a regular basis, usually twice a week or weekly for 50 minute sessions (preferably at the same time of day and on the same day or days of the week) and in return the individual agrees not to lose any more weight. The aim of this is to try to establish a safe and contained therapeutic situation which is encouraged both by the individual opting into it and also by her feeling that, although body weight is not *un*important, it is not going to be the central focus of sessions. Often, she may have had previous experiences where she felt that the main focus of concern was whether or not she had gained the requisite poundage that week. In addition, being asked only to maintain her weight in the first instance may be experienced with feelings of relief. Hence, the individual would not be weighed, nor would a 'target weight' be set for her.

Early on, information is provided about the behavior of dieting and also about the various health risks connected with self-starvation, with vomitting and with laxative abuse (when relevant). Nutritional and dietary education is again included as well as information about exercise, behavioral strategies and practical supports found to be effective in facilitating gradual and steady gain of body weight. More often than not, the individual knows a lot of this already. The aim is not to preach or prescribe weight-gaining diets, but again to work on an individualized basis, giving relevant information and accounting for likes and dislikes, food fears and food fads, and so forth.

As the therapeutic relationship is established, an integrated psychotherapy evolves which is not structured, rushed or time-tabled. Cognitive, emotional and interpersonal factors emerge in the client's own time and in her own way. In the end the goal for the client is to enable her to construct for herself her own sense of worth and identity, without removing her fragile sense of self-control but, rather, supporting her in what she chooses to do for herself.

The importance of cognitive factors has been widely recognized by many people in this field, wherein cognitions require a careful re-evaluation by the individual herself. She enters therapy with what she believes to be her reality and this should not be deconstructed for her, especially when it is often rooted in socially promulgated half-truths. A fear of becoming obese if she relinquishes her control over her food and hence a fear of the social consequences of that potential obesity, is not actually so unreal. Obesity *is* both stigmatized and marginalized in this society and it can be unhealthy. It is also true that some individuals who have suffered self-starvation have gone on to experience both binge-eating and subsequent overweight. Thus, enabling an individual to re-evaluate her thoughts about her body shape requires a realistic acknowledgement of the wider social situation as well as her own individual circumstances (Garner and Garfinkel, 1980).

Cognitions about particular foods, the notorious 'good food' and 'bad food' lists owned by many individuals, are perhaps easier for the individual to view differently. This is because, despite the mass media bombardment of messages about what to eat and what not to eat, the individual may often have taken on board messages which were not only not targeted for her but which for her may prove counter-productive. In this sense, she may have adopted the classic all or nothing, dichotomous pattern of thinking mistakes. If she can be enabled to accept that consuming small amounts of high energy foods is fine, then all that remains very often is to help her to construct situations for herself where she can experiment with eating these small quantities, without her feeling that once she starts she won't be able to stop.

Throughout all this, the individual needs to know that the therapist is aware of the conflicts between thoughts and feelings that are going on for the individual. Self-statements such as "I know I should be heavier, but I can't help *feeling* big" and "I know one chocolate won't make me fat, but I feel it in my stomach for hours afterwards" frequently occur.

Emotional expression varies tremendously, from those who deny their feelings early on to those whose pain and anger very quickly emerge. It is vital to facilitate emotional expression and the therapist who can accept and encourage the individual's feelings to emerge in sessions can provide an environment where emotions can be experienced and their origins and consequences can be explored.

Often anger has been turned inwards because the individual cannot cope with the idea of feeling angry towards somebody she wants to love unconditionally. Parents and partners may have been idealized in such a way that they are experienced as unreachable. Social pressures to conform to a particular shape or weight may be experienced as rules which go unchallenged. One part of the therapeutic *raison d'etre* is to enable the individual to understand the interpersonal motivations underlying her problems.

A behavioral or even a purely cognitive approach is unlikely in isolation to enable individuals to escape fully from their self-destructive behavior. For some, their self-starvation may feel like the only way in which they can communicate with their family and the society around them, the only way they can say "I'm here, I'm lonely, I have needs, and I want you to satisfy them". Individuals may experience conflicts between wanting to idealize their parents and, at the same time, feeling very angry with them. Identifying the reasons for this can enable individuals to communicate with them in different and more effective ways, to accept their shortcomings, to ask them for some emotional nurturance and also to look outside their families as well as within themselves for the satisfaction of needs they might now be able to allow themselves to have. Other interpersonal influences might include the peer and social pressures experienced by some individuals when younger as a consequence of being slightly overweight, the euphemistic 'puppy fat', or as a consequence of the confusion felt about the meaning of being an adult female and about what role or roles to adopt. Such issues may emerge particularly in the case of a mother who has adopted a domestic role when current expectations often point in the direction of educational achievement and career.

In the context of the above, the value of group-based interventions has increasingly been acknowledged. These can be either facilitated by a professional or be of a 'self-help' nature. Open groups might be conducted for individuals who are emerging from these difficulties and these can act as supportive stepping stones towards their fuller empowerment. A variety of skills-based groups, such as assertion training, may be needed for people who feel they want to be able to enhance skills which may not have been fully acquired. Also, physiotherapy can enable an individual to come to terms with a body she may fear, to cope with gaining weight, and with regard to engaging in appropriate rather than excessive exercise.

CONCLUSIONS

Such an approach as the one described above provides a framework of components to draw upon, components aimed at enabling and empowering women in distress. It differs fundamentally from approaches which involve the imposition of a particular 'treatment' upon the individual. As we contended earlier, however, such an approach is not in itself sufficient. What is also required is change on a wider scale, change which would encompass social attitudes and which would have a preventative impact upon the incidence of dieting distress and 'eating disorders'. It may be that more needs to be done in schools, in order to counter the impact of media pressures and to identify problems in the early stages. Perhaps we also need, however, to be helping potential parents more. Women need to be campaigning against industries who profit from the promulgation of thin as the ideal and from the marketing of 'diet' products where 90 percent of body weight lost is re-gained and 5 percent of the female population experience self-starvation or the vicious cycle of binge-eating and vomitting and/or laxative abuse.

Given the context in which women live in Western societies at the present time, it is perhaps surprising not that 'eating disorders' exist, but rather that they are not far more widespread. It is a reflection of women's strength and stamina that they do not succumb more to the socio-cultural and political pressures upon them. At a time when women are increasingly empowering themselves, perhaps there is an opportunity for significant cultural shifts to begin to take place which will free them from the destructive coupling of self-esteem with food consumption and body image.

FURTHER READING

Chermin, K. (1985). *The hungry self. Women, eating and identity*. London: Virago.
Crisp, A.H. (1980). *Anorexia nervosa: Let me be*. London: Academic Press.
Orbach, S. (1982). *Fat is a feminist issue* 2. London: Hamlyn Paperbacks.

9

WOMEN AND DEPRESSION

RAYMOND COCHRANE

School of Psychology, The University of Birmingham, Edgbaston, Birmingham B15 2TT, UK

In this chapter some of the evidence concerning gender differences in the rate of depressive disorders in England will be reviewed and an examination made of some of the explanations that have been put forward to account for these differences in terms of how well each of them fit the data that are available.

The starting point for this analysis is the comparison of male and female mental hospitalization rates shown in Table 9.1. These data are completely congruent with those produced by many other researchers in England and in several other countries. They show that, overall, women are about 40 percent more likely to be admitted to a mental hospital each year than are men. The differential in first admission rates is less than this at about 30 percent; and slightly more than the overall figure for re-admissions to hospital after first admission, where the female excess reached 43 percent in 1981. Given that the gender ratio differences between all, first, and re-admissions is relatively small, only 'all admissions' will be referred to in future as these, arguably, are the best index of the number of people receiving inpatient treatment in any one year.

It is important to note that the data in Table 9.1 are unstandardized other than being sex-specific. There are two important variables to take into consideration when trying to understand these data: age and diagnosis. In England, as elsewhere, rates of mental hospitalization rise rapidly in the elderly population, reaching a figure of over 1,000 per 100,000 for those over 75 years old: in this age group women outnumber men by two to one due to their greater longevity. Thus, it is necessary to age-standardize the admission figures to avoid age differences in the at-risk population distorting the male:female comparison. When this is done the all-admission rate differential reduces to 132 women for every 100 men in 1981 (compared to 140:100 for the unstandardized data).

Turning to diagnostic differences in the mental hospital admission patterns of men and women it is clear that the diagnosis which contributes most to the higher overall

TABLE 9.1
Mental hospital admission rates for England, 1981.

Admission	Rate per 100,000 population		Female rate as percent of male rate
	Females	Males	
First admission	130	99	131
Re-admission	341	238	143
All admissions	471	337	140

rate of admission for women is depression (which here includes the diagnoses of affective psychoses, depressive disorders, and neurotic depression). In this category the age-adjusted female rate is almost twice the male rate and it is also by far the largest single cause of mental hospital admissions, accounting for almost one in every two female admissions and one in every three male admissions. Women also outnumber men in the residual neurosis category, but this is a relatively small group, as are the diagnostic categories of schizophrenia and alcohol and drug related admissions where men outnumber women (Table 9.2). The pattern is very similar in North America. McGrath *et al.* (1990) and Nolen-Hoeksema (1987) have both recently conducted extensive reviews of the literature on gender differences in depression and came to the same conclusion: the average male:female ratio for the prevalence of depression is close

TABLE 9.2
Age adjusted, sexspecific sites of all admissions to mental hospitals in England, 1981.

Diagnostic Cate	Rate per 100,000 population		Female rate as percent of male rate
	Females	Males	
Schizophrenia and Paranoia	62	65	95
Depression (a)	200	101	198
Neuroses (b)	21	11	190
Personality and behaviour disorder	36	30	120
Alcohol and Drug related disorders	25	51	49
Other diagnoses (c)	111	88	126
All diagnoses	455	346	132

(a) Includes affective psychoses, depressive disorder and neurotic depression.
(b) Excludes neurotic depression.
(c) Includes senility, organic disorders, retardation, undiagnosed cases, and non-psychiatric admissions.

to 1:2. A male to female ratio of lifetime prevalence of depression of 1:2.2 has been reported from Puerto Rico (Canino *et al.*, 1987).

The basic gender difference in treated mental illness rates is a difference in the rates of depression.

EXPLANATIONS

There are almost as many explanations for these data as there are epidemiologists and others who have tried to account for them, but they can be broken down into six categories of explanation which are not, of course, mutually exclusive.

1. Treated Prevalence Does Not Reflect True Incidence

It is widely acknowledged that treated prevalence, especially when based on mental hospital in-patient statistics, considerably under-represent true incidence rates – indeed they only represent the proverbial tip of the iceberg. This would not be a serious problem in this context if it could be assumed that the ratio of treated to untreated cases were the same for both sexes – we could simply scale-up the figures to obtain a more veridical estimate of the real prevalence of depression. Unfortunately, it is not possible to make this assumption as no firm evidence for it (or against it) exists. Some attempts to examine the relationship between true prevalence and treated prevalence seem to indicate that the latter *underestimates* gender differences in true prevalence ie. women are *less* likely to be referred and treated at the same level of psychological distress than are men (Goldberg and Huxley, 1980).

What can be said with more certainty is that women in England have higher rates of depression than do men whether this indexed by all types of contact with services (outpatients, in-patients, and family doctors etc.), use of antidepressant medications, or through the measurement of depressive symptomatology in random samples of the non-hospitalized population. In one study that is representative of many, many others, Cochrane and Stopes-Roe (1981) found significantly higher levels of self-reported depressive symptoms among a random sample of women than from an equivalent sample of men. This study will be considered again later in this chapter. North American research has also confirmed that gender differences in rates of depression are not confined to only those cases that present for treatment, but are also to be found among untreated cases (McGrath *et al.*, 1990).

Thus the differences in treated prevalence rates cannot be dismissed as an artefact produced by biases in admission statistics nor even by the possibility that women have a lower threshold for seeking treatment than do men.

2. Biological Differences

The most widely accepted popular explanation for gender differences in proneness to depression is that women are innately more emotional than men and, therefore, more prone to emotional upsets. At first glance this is a reasonable proposition because, quite probably, there are differences between the emotional responsiveness of men and women at any particular point in time. For biological explanations to be considered valid, however, the difference between the sexes should, a) show consistency across different social categories and b) ultimately some sex-linked mechanisms for the basis of the biological differences would have to be demonstrated.

On the first of these criteria – consistency across social categories – the biological explanation apparently runs into trouble when marital status is added as a variable to the analysis. In Table 9.3 the data on the treated prevalence of depression in England in 1981 are broken down by the legal marital category to which the patients belonged at the time of their admission. There are three points of interest to note from this table. First, the absolute rates for both men and women vary considerably with marital category. Being married was associated with low relative risk for both sexes. These age-standardized data reveal that divorced women were 3.7 times more likely to be treated for depression than were married women (this ratio rises to 6.2:1 for divorced:married men). Second, widowed and divorced men were conspicuously more likely to be depressed than were single or married women. Third, the greater vulnerability of women than men to depression varied considerably with marital category. Only among the married is the large excess of women over men found. Although the married of both sexes have the lowest level of depression, by far the largest proportion of the adult population is, in fact, married (see Cochrane, 1988). Thus the higher rate of depression found among married women than among married men tends to mask the equally important observation that women have lower rates of depression than do men in the single, widowed and divorced categories.

On the surface it seems that putative biological differences between men and women cannot account for the large variations in the relative risk of depression produced by moving from one socially defined category to another. However, Gater *et al.* (1989) have recently produced a new analysis introducing the additional variable of parity into the explanation of gender differences in one form of depression. Beginning with the observation that the differences between men and women are greatest during the female child bearing years, they showed that women who had borne children had a much greater treated incidence rate for affective psychosis than did non-parous women *whether or not they were married.* In fact in this study it was only women who had given birth to children who had a higher risk than men: marital status added nothing to the predictive power of parity. Gater *et al.* suggest that the most parsimonious explanation for their findings is that a biological mechanism is switched on during pregnancy or child bearing which leaves parous women at greater risk of affective psychosis for most of the rest of their lives. They do, however, acknowledge that the

TABLE 9.3

Age adjusted, sex specific, rates for all admissions to mental hospitals with a diagnosis of depression (a) in England, 1981 by marital status.

Marital Status	Rates per 100,000 population		Female rate as percent of male rate
	Females	Males	
Single	269	185	145
Married	160	70	229
Widowed	420	341	123
Divorced	599	432	139

(a) Includes affective psychoses, depressive disorders and neurotic depression.

same effect could be produced by the social circumstance of motherhood – a point to which I will return later.

Merikangas *et al.* (1985) tested the possibility that there were sex-linked genetic factors that might account for gender differences in depression by looking at the relative risk for depression in the male and female relatives of depressed patients of both sexes. No evidence to support the genetic hypothesis was found.

Although various other biological mechanisms which may cause sex differences in psychological state, particularly depression, have been suggested – such as pre-menstrual tension, the immediate effects of childbirth, the menopause, and even the use of oral contraceptives, these in fact are very unlikely to account for the large differences found in the rates of depression between the two sexes. In a thorough review of biological agents which could possibly influence proneness to depression Weissman and Klerman (1977) concluded that "while some portion of the sex differences in depression, probably during the child bearing years may be explained endocrinologically, this factor is not sufficient to account for the large differences" (p. 106). They found, for example, that the effect of the menopause on a woman's psychological state was itself socially mediated: women who are led to believe that the menopause may be associated with emotional upsets find that this becomes a self-fulfilling prophecy. There is no hard evidence that the menopause produces a direct effect on psychological functioning.

Similarly with post-partum depression, it is widely acknowledged that a significanct proportion of women become depressed following the birth of a baby. What is not clear, however, is the actual extent, severity, nature, course and outcome of these depressive episodes. The most careful studies report incidence rates of between 6 and 20 percent, but only a small fraction of the women who experience depression at this time seek treatment (Hopkins *et al.*, 1984). Very few studies have compared the incidence of depression (however defined) in women who have given birth recently and in women of similar age and social circumstance who have not. Cooper *et al.* (1988) recently reported a meticulously careful study of the prevalence of depression prior to childbirth when 6 percent of women were affected and shortly after childbirth when the figure was 8.7 percent. Of a sample of non-pregnant women of the same age, 9.9 percent met the definition of being depressed used in this study. Thus, having recently given birth to a child did not increase a woman's risk of becoming depressed, so logically cannot be used as an explanation of the higher rates found for women than for men.

So far, then, no biological mechanism has been positively identified which could account for sex differences in depression, although a hypothetical link to childbearing has been posited.

3. Long-term Effects of Child Abuse

Child abuse, both physical and sexual, has recently become a major field of psychological investigation and it could have some bearing on the elevated risk for depression shown by adult women. The argument depends on bringing together two strands of research on child abuse – epidemiology and outcome studies. It is now widely documented that child abuse in one form or another is far from uncommon. Estimates of the proportion of children affected depend on methodology and the definitions of abuse used, but in England they range from a low figure of 10 percent to figures as high as 46 percent (Search, 1988). In the US, estimates range from under 5 percent to over 50 percent (Starr *et al*. 1990). In every study from which data are available for boys and girls separately, the rate of abuse of girls is much higher, especially in the case of sexual abuse. The actual ratio found varies from between 1.5:1 to 4.5:1 depending on the study (Alter-Reid *et al*., 1986; Search, 1988).

The second aspect of child abuse which is relevant is the equally strong evidence that when abused children grow up they suffer adverse psychological consequences as a result of the abuse and that this frequently manifests itself as depression. Again figures vary from study to study, but victims of child abuse are at least twice as likely to suffer clinical depression in adulthood as are non-victims (Becker *et al*., 1983; Gold, 1986; Search, 1988). Looked at another way, Bryer *et al*. (1987) found that over 70 percent of a consecutive cohort of depressed patients admitted to a hospital in Massachusetts had been abused as children.

Putting these figures together produces a potent argument to account for sex differences in depression: child abuse happens much more often to girls than to boys and abuse is heavily implicated as an etiological agent in depression. Thus, child abuse could be sufficiently widespread in Britain to account for the fact that twice as many women as men are treated for depression in mental hospitals every year.

4. Gender-role Socialisation Produces Increased Female Vulnerability

There are a number of factors in the different identities and roles created by society for women and men and indeed in the power relationships between the two sexes, which may also provide an explanation for sex differences in rates of depression.

Sex discrimination has become a well documented and researched phenomenon in western societies. It is obviously true that in many areas of employment (job opportunities, relative remuneration and promotion prospects for example) and in personal relationships, women are often at a disadvantage compared to men. It would be surprising indeed if the institutionalized inequality produced by social definitions did not exact a psychological price upon the disadvantaged group.

Probably just as important as the direct effects of sex discrimination on mental health, however, are the equally powerful effects of gender role definition which underlie these structural inequalities. Traditional gender role definitions are based on the notion of complementarily between men and women: for example men are supposed to be active and forceful while women are supposed to be more passive and submissive. However, it is obvious, even from a cursory examination of the traits traditionally considered appropriate for men and women, that the assignment of these traits has not been without bias. "Since men hold the power and authority, women are rewarded for developing a set of psychological characteristics that accommodate to and please men. Such traits – submissiveness, compliance, passivity, helplessness, weakness – have been encouraged in women and incorporated into some prevalent psychological theories in which they are defined as innate or inevitable characteristics of women." (Carmen *et al*., 1981, p. 1321).

In a variety of contexts women who accept, or who are forced to accept, traditional sex role definitions will experience a relatively low capacity to influence their environment and to control their own lives. Women are more likely to be conditioned to define themselves in terms of their ability to attract a spouse and to achieve their own identities vicariously through the achievements of their husbands. These factors in women's lives may very well contribute to the development of learned helplessness which Seligman (1975) and others have suggested is a precursor of clinical depression. To the extent that the learned helplessness hypothesis holds water, then, their relatively low capacity to influence their own psychological outcomes compared to men will make women significantly more vulnerable to depression.

Gender role socialization may also affect the way in which psychological problems manifest themselves in men and women. Warren (1983) has made a persuasive case that depression is much more uncomfortable for men that for women as it is much more discrepant with the masculine stereotype than the feminine stereotype. The former includes competence, toughness and the avoidance of anything that smacks of femininity, while depression includes manifestations of helplessness, weakness and vulnerability and emotional expressiveness, perhaps even crying, which are traditionally associated with femininity, not masculinity. While women may be willing to admit to depressive affect and seek social and professional support and hence risk becoming identified as depressed, men will find other outlets for problems of adjustment which are more congruent with their self image – heavy drinking for example, which is much more common among men. A case could also be made that anti-depressive medication makes patients (both men and women) more 'feminine' in the sense that it induces a degree of passivity and acquiescence, while alcohol has a 'masculinizing' effect, producing self-confidence and aggression.

All these arguments in favor of socialization differences producing the higher rates of depression in women are undermined to some extent by the marital status, parity and age effects already referred to. There must be some factors in addition to being brought up as a boy or a girl influencing vulnerability to depression.

5. Specific Aspects of the Adult Female Role are Pathonomic

It seems that neither biological explanations nor explanations based upon gender role socialization can cope with all the types of data which have been produced relevant to understanding gender differences in depression. Attention has turned increasingly to an examination of what factors occur in the middle years of women's lives which produce the exaggeration of differences in rates of depression compared to men (see Figure 9.1). The obvious constellation of events during this life cycle stage is: marriage-childbearing-motherhood. Gater *et al.* (1989) have shown that having children is strongly predictive of higher risk of depression for women (but not for men) but were unable to determine whether this was a biological effect or a result of the social circumstances of motherhood. Typically, having children produces a considerable change in the life-style of women and the changes are much more fundamental and far reaching that they are for fathers. Mothers still usually assume prime responsibility for most aspects of child care and the other domestic functions indirectly associated with child care – cleaning, cooking, washing, etc. Some sociologists have considered that these activities may, in themselves, be a cause of depression (eg. Gove, 1972, 1984; Gove and Tudor, 1973) but increasingly attention has turned to the effects of not having paid employment outside the home as a consequence of taking on the role of full-time housewife and mother.

Early evidence which drew attention to this factor was provided in the well known study of depression in women by Brown and Harris (1978). They interviewed over 400 women living in London and found that between 20 and 40 percent of their sample had

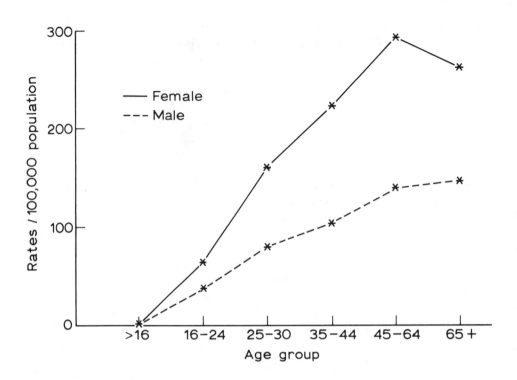

FIGURE 9.1 Age-specific rates for depression—all admissions, England, 1981.

experienced some psychological problems during the previous year which approached clinical levels of severity. Of these, the great majority turned out to be cases of depression which were often associated with some severe stress usually revolving around a loss of an important person by separation or death. However, as is to be expected, there were a number of other women in the sample who had experienced a serious stressful episode in the same period but who did not become depressed. Brown and Harris identified four factors in a woman's life which made her more vulnerable to the effects of stress and therefore liable to become depressed. These factors included having several young children to care for and not having paid employment outside the home. Although paid employment did not provide as much protection against the effects of stress, in the sense of preventing stress from producing depression, as having an intimate and confiding relationship with someone else, in the absence of such a relationship, having a job almost halved the number of women who became depressed following a severe life event.

The effect of not having a job can be just as debilitating for men as for women, but it is married women with children who are most likely to be out of the labor market. In 1984 nearly 90 percent of men in England were economically active compared to less than 50 percent of married women (Social Trends, 1986). Thus, substantially more married women were 'unprotected' by paid employment than were men.

Cochrane and Stopes-Roe, (1980, 1981) assessed random community samples of men and women with a depression inventory. Overall, women had significantly higher scored than did men (Table 9.4). When employment status was controlled for, however,

TABLE 9.4
Average depression scale scores in random community samples by gender and
employment status.

	Female		Male		
	N	$\overline{X}$	N	$\overline{X}$	p <
Total	109	3.1	150	2.4	0.05
Employed	55	2.1	126	2.1	NS
Not employed	54	4.2	24	4.2	NS
p <		0.01		0.01	

there were no differences between the sexes: working women had identical scores to working men; non-employed women had identical scores to non-employed men. For both sexes the non-employed had significantly higher mean scores than did the employed, but as there were proportionately more non-employed women, the average score for all women was elevated above that for all men. A multiple regression analysis on these data showed that for both women and men separately, employment status was by far the best predictor of psychological well-being, with other variables adding relatively little to the predictive power of having paid employment.

In fact the evidence that shows that paid employment is as important to the psychological well-being of women as it is for men is extremely strong (eg. Tennant *et al.*, 1982; Thoits, 1986), but there has also been the suggestion that a married woman who works outside the home may experience another form of psychological stress resulting from role conflicts, especially if she is the mother of young children (eg. Warr and Parry, 1982). This stress could derive both from the physical demands on her time and energy made by the twin responsibilities of children and career and from a fear that she might not be fulfilling either role (especially the maternal role) adequately.

This has led to the concept of 'role overload', which is produced by occupying too many roles, or roles that are in some crucial way incompatible, which, it is hypothesized, in turn leads to stress and hence to illness. However, the evidence has not been kind to this concept. In fact, so overwhelmingly negative has been the evidence and it should be said, so strong the prevailing social attitudes of those involved in researching this topic, that the role overload concept has been completely reversed and the 'multiple role' hypothesis has taken its place (Barnett and Baruch, 1985). This posits that the more roles occupied the better, in health terms. There is no inevitable conflict between roles, and the positive gains from each role occupied cumulate to produce increments in well-being and defences against depression (Thoits, 1986; Barnett and Baruch, 1985; Kandel *et al.*, 1985; Froberg *et al.*, 1986).

6. Depression as a Coping Strategy for Women

So far, the common assumption has been made that the manifestation of depression is inevitably a sign of psychopathology and an indication of hopelessness and despair – a form of giving up. I have argued before (Cochrane and Sobol, 1980) that depression (and other forms of 'mental illness') may also be seen as a positive coping response in

TABLE 9.5
Hierarchy of coping resources (From *more* to *less* socially desirable).

Response to stress	Example	More available to men or women?
Intrapsychic defences	Self esteem, mastery, self deception	Men
Stress opposing experiences	Success, promotion, achievement, social recognition, positive affect balance	Men
Initimate social	Spouse, lover, parent	Men
Less intimate social support	Workmate, friend relative	Equal?
Substance abuse	Alcohol, drugs	Men
Self-harm	Overdosing, cutting	Women
Psychophysiological symptoms	Anxiety, crying, appetite loss, nervousness	Women
Sanctioned mental illness	Depression	Women

certain circumstances. Now, no one would choose to become depressed if they had alternative ways of coping with their problems of living which were more socially and personally acceptable and also effective. The generally accepted view is that depression develops when the coping resources available to a person are exhausted by the continued presence of stresses and strains. However, sometimes depression might not be a pathological response to unbearable stress but a valuable and adaptive reaction to stress that is used when other types of response are either not available or, if they are available, have been tried and seen to fail. Some significant part of the variability in the incidence of depression between the sexes may be accounted for by the differential availability of other coping resources to men and women.

Table 9.5 contains a list of ways of coping with stress which have been organized according to an estimate of their social desirability. The third column of the table suggests whether men or women are more likely to have access to each kind of coping strategy, although this too reflects a subjective judgement. Individual variations within each sex will mean that not all men, nor all women, will have access to these coping resources. What it is intended to imply is that a *higher proportion* of men or women will be able to respond in this way than members of the other gender.

The first four coping resources listed in the table are all more or less socially acceptable ways of trying to deal with the effects of stress. They are techniques which are not only looked upon in a positive light but they are often deliberately inculcated by psychologists and social workers as coping skills where they believe these to be lacking. The remainder of the responses contained in the Table reflect what is often considered to be deviant behavior of a more or less serious kind. The nature of the deviance entered into at each stage will itself be heavily influenced by gender and other social characteristics.

Men are much more likely than women to respond to incipient psychological problems with heavy drinking and other forms of drug abuse. This is particularly true of less educated men who may be less likely to have sophisticated psychological explanations for their own feelings of frustration available to them than their more educated middle-class counterparts. Heavy alcohol use has also been analyzed as a coping strategy (Davis *et al.*, 1974). An equivalent female form of deviant behavior is deliberate self harm in the form of drug overdosing which is often a unilateral attempt to alter a social situation. Although overdoses are taken by people of all ages and both sexes, it is a behavior that, in Britain at least, is very heavily concentrated among young, working-class women.

It is at the next level in the hierarchy that the gradual progress of the person towards fully formed and recognized depression may begin. The first stage will be the development of symptoms which are usually seen as a result of intolerable stress which cannot be handled properly. In line with the argument being made here, however, they may also be interpreted as genuine attempts at adaptation. The occurrence and persistence of psychological symptoms may indeed serve positive functions for the person affected. In much the same way as the symptoms of physical illness are sometimes effective in changing a situation, or the social definitions associated with that situation, so may psychological symptoms be instrumentally effective.

Particularly in the case of women, for whom the admission of psychological symptoms is less likely to be seen as a sign of weakness, this may be one of the few forms of influence open to them inside certain relationships – the only way of dealing with an otherwise intractable situation. Depression is seen by some as a way of using psychological symptoms to persuade others to satisfy the depressed person's goals which may be to gain the support or subjugation of other people, for example. Bonime (1976) analyzed depression as a way of life developed by some people to wring the most out of others by exploiting their generosity and sense of responsibility. This is done by making sure that other people are fully aware of the extent of the patient's depressive symptoms and are affected by them. Some people may, Bonime suggests, use their depression to gain an advantage in a relationship that they could not otherwise achieve through manipulation of their relatives' sense of guilt and concern, either consciously or unconsciously. In either event they are able, at least for some time, to get their own way in certain matters. Of course, this is a high risk strategy as the caregiver might get tired of being placed in this uncomfortable position and react by totally withdrawing support.

Any adaptive advantage conveyed by the development of psychological symptoms will be multiplied by having a formal recognition that illness exists. In our society, illness certified as such by a doctor confers a very particular status on the person. This status may be deliberately sought and used by a much larger number of people than is customarily recognised. The consequences of illness diagnosis will be particularly attractive to those who lack the resources to manage their lives in other ways. Again women, particularly those with poor marriage, or marital-type relationships, who are perhaps unable to communicate their difficulties directly with their partner are most likely to fall into this category; even more so if they are not at work and, therefore, do not have access to alternative coping mechanisms such as those described above.

The ultimate consequence of the sick role is, of course, admission to a hospital. Although most people would consider a sojourn in a mental hospital as an experience to be avoided at any cost, there are undoubtedly some people who gain considerable benefit from such an episode in their lives. I do not here mean people who receive particularly effective treatment for their condition, but rather those who manage to alter their social situation dramatically by a period of hospitalization.

Although it is not being suggested that this is the only reason for their higher rates of inpatient treatment, statistics consistently bear out the fact that women and also other disadvantaged groups, (eg. the poor, the isolated, the unemployed, the homeless, the elderly, and some minority ethnic groups) are more likely to be referred for inpatient treatment than other social groups (Cochrane, 1983). The argument here is that this reflects the lack of alternative coping resources at least as much as it reflects the natural tendency to depression, or excessive stress, borne by some women in particular situations.

CONCLUSION

The various explanations offerred for the higher incidence of depression found among women than among men are not, of course, mutually exclusive. They may well all contribute to any satisfactory and complete explanation. Having said that, it does seem that the most powerful clues to the particular vulnerability of women to depression lie in the unique constellation of circumstances surrounding the experience of motherhood and child care – what it gives to women and what it takes away.

FURTHER READING

Cochrane, R. (1983). *The social creation of mental illness*. London: Longmans.

Miles, A. (1988). *Women and mental illness: The social context of female neuroses*. Brighton: Wheatsheaf.

Travis, C.B. (1988). *Women and health psychology: Mental health issues*. Hillsdale, New Jersey: Erlbaum.

10

MEDICAL SCREENING FOR WOMEN

GILLIAN McILWAINE

Greater Glasgow Health Board, Department of Public Health, Glasgow Royal Maternity Hospital, Rottenrow, Glasgow G4 0NA, UK

During this century there have been striking advances in medical knowledge and technology which have contributed to increased life expectancy as well as greater expectations by the public of what medicine can achieve. A baby girl born today is likely to live for at least 76 years compared to only 50 years if she had been born at the beginning of the century. Much of this improvement has occurred because of the considerable reduction in mortality during infancy and childhood. Childbirth is now relatively safe for women and a maternal death is fortunately a very rare event. At the Glasgow Royal Maternity Hospital, for instance (where I work), which was opened in 1834, one in 50 mothers died in childbirth in the 1920s, compared with a rate of one death in 18,000 births today. There are many factors which have contributed to this improvement, but the availability of antenatal screening for all women has obviously played a part. One of the main aims of this care is to detect a problem which might affect the mother or her unborn child at an early stage so that treatment can be instituted and the best possible outcome achieved.

WHAT IS SCREENING?

The concept of screening in health care "that is, actively seeking to identify a disease or predisease condition in people who are presumed and presume themselves to be healthy" – is one that has now wide acceptance in our society (Holland and Stewart, 1990). To many it may seem perverse to look for problems: "never trouble trouble, until trouble troubles you," as the old saying goes. Others feel that we must do all we can, whatever the cost to reduce the incidence of the disease.

In 1968, Wilson and Junger, in a World Health Organisation Public Health paper, laid down the criteria which should be considered when a screening programme is being proposed. These criteria still stand today and are as follows:

The condition sought should be an important health problem; there should be an accepted treatment for the patient with the recognized disease; facilities for treatment and diagnosis should be available; there should be a recognizable latent or early symptomatic stage and a suitable test or examination; the test should be acceptable to the population; the natural history of the disease, including latent and declared disease, should be adequately understood; there should be an agreed policy on whom to treat as patients; the cost of case-finding (including diagnosis and treatment of patients diagnosed) should be economically balanced in relation to possible expenditure on medical care as a whole; case-finding should be a continuing process and not a 'once for all' project.

Holland and Stewart (1990) have collapsed these principles into four categories – condition, diagnosis, treatment and cost.

CAN SCREENING DO HARM?

While the motives behind screening programmes are certainly well intentioned, it is still necessary to pose the question "can screening do harm?" Inviting a woman (or man or child) to come for a screening test is different from other aspects of medical care in that in this instance, the provider of care is offering to look for a potential problem, which at the time of screening is not causing any trouble. Accordingly, the client undergoing screening differs from the person seeking treatment for a known condition or problem. It should, therefore, be imperative that in offering a screening test, no harm will be done to the individual. The benefits and disadvantages of the screening test must be considered from both the physical and psychological point of view. This is well demonstrated in the publication produced by the UK Cancer Research Campaign for primary care doctors (Austoker *et al.*, 1989) explaining the rationale behind the national breast screening programme that was introduced in 1988 for British women aged 50–64 years of age (Forrest, 1986). In this booklet the physical and psychological benefits and disadvantages of a screening test are summarized.

The possible benefits are listed as life years gained for those with curable cancer and avoidance of morbidity related to radical treatment. The disadvantages are the complications resulting from the screening test itself (eg. bruising following a blood test). There is also extended morbidity if the prognosis is unaltered, as well as the possibility of over diagnosis, resulting in women receiving unnecessary treatment for lesions which otherwise might have regressed spontaneously.

On the psychological side, the benefits can be summarized as: reassurance in those where cancer is not present; reassurance that the disease is at a very early stage; possible psychological advantages of avoiding radical treatment. The disadvantages include fear of being found to have cancer when invited for screening; false reassurance for those whose cancer goes undetected (false negative); and a longer period of anxiety for those who have an incurable disease or non-progressive cancer.

SCREENING PROGRAMMES FOR WOMEN

There are now a umber of screening programmes available for women, ranging from a care package, such as antenatal care, to the detection of a specific abnormality such as carcinoma of the breast. In this section I will concentrate on antenatal care and screening tests for women introduced to reduce death from cancer.

Antenatal care

The pattern of antenatal care is remarkably similar throughout the Western world. Antenatal care consists of a number of screening tests for the mother and the baby. They include blood pressure measurement and urinalysis to detect signs of pregnancy induced hypertension, a serious condition, which in extreme form may endanger the life of the mother and her unborn child. Women are always screened for anaemia and the presence of antibodies in the blood (eg. rhesus antibody) which may affect the baby.

Most women also have an ultrasound scan around 18 weeks gestation to assess the size of the baby and to determine whether there is any sign of neural tube abnormality such as spina bifida or anencephaly. Writing about ultrasound in *Effective Care in Pregnancy and Childbirth*, Neilson and Grant (1990) state that systematic attention has not been paid to women's reactions to ultrasonography during pregnancy and that the studies that have been conducted have included only women with normal pregnancies. Such studies have shown that women value an ultrasound examination early in pregnancy, because it confirms the reality of the pregnancy and is often followed by a reduction in anxiety and an increase in confidence. The examination can have negative effects however, arising from a lack of communication between the ultrasonographer and the women and this may, on occasion, nullify its potentially beneficial psychological effects. The value of good communication, Neilson and Grant (1990) contend, has been demonstrated in four randomized controlled trials. In one trial there was some suggestion that when women were given feedback they were likely to reduce cigarette smoking and alcohol consumption. However, this reduction was not found in other trials and was anyway only a short term effect.

The increasing medicalization of pregnancy and the transfer of power from women to their medical carers continues to be a matter of controversy. Evidence is now emerging that part of antenatal care concerned with aspects of social support, such as information giving, health education, counselling and more positive care giving, is associated with significant benefits: a reduction in the amount of drugs used for pain relief in labor; a reduction in the risk of prolonged labor; and reductions in the risk of instrumental delivery, maternal anxiety and postnatal depression (Elbourne *et al.*, 1990).

Screening tests are also offered to the mother during pregnancy to detect abnormality in the fetus, such as Downs Syndrome or a neural tube defect. There is a large literature about the screening for fetal abnormality and this is discussed further in Chapter 3.

Early cancer detection

Cancer is the most frequent cause of premature death in women in the Western world. In Scotland in 1990 there were 4880 deaths in women between 25 and 64 years of age, 43.7 percent of which were due to cancer (Registrar General Scotland, 1990).

When individual cancers are reviewed in the under 65 years age group, breast cancer is the commonest cancer in Scottish women accounting for 502 deaths, followed by lung cancer which accounted for 443 deaths. When all ages are considered, lung cancer causes most cancer deaths in Scottish women. Finally, there were 80 deaths from cervical cancer in women under 65 years of age in Scotland.

Screening aims to detect presymptomatic cancer at a stage in its natural history at which treatment will arrest its progression. A clear answer as to whether or not screening is worthwhile is only available for four cancer sites – cervix, breast, lung and testes (Royal College of Physicians, 1991). The considered conclusion is that screening is worthwhile for cervix and breast, but not for lung (this should be dealt with by primary prevention, by curtailing cigarette smoking) or testes where it is regarded as unnecessary because chemotherapy now achieves cure rates of 90 percent or more, even in advanced cases.

Screening for pre-cancer of the cervix

The question is often asked, given the relatively low rates of mortality, why so much attention and press coverage is given to screening for cervical cancer? The answer is simple. Until recently, cervical cancer was the only cancer which could be detected at a pre-cancerous stage by a simple screening test with major benefit because of effective treatment. In other words, it fits nearly all of the criteria laid down by Wilson and Junger, described earlier in this chapter.

Cervical cancer accounts for 2,000 deaths in British women each year, 17 percent of whom are less than 45 years of age. The cause of the disease is not fully understood, but all the evidence to date points to a viral infection. The herpes and wart viruses have both been implicated but the precise agent is yet to be unambiguously identified. The risk of developing cervical cancer increases if intercourse begins at a young age, if a sexually transmitted disease is present and if the woman or her partner has had a large number of sexual partners (Hobbs *et al.*, 1985).

In the 1940s in America, Papanicolaou and Trout (1943) devised a simple test which removed cells from the uterine cervix. Employing this test it was not only possible to distinguish normal and cancerous cells, but also to identify cells in varying stages of change (from mild to severe). A pre-cancerous change could therefore be identified and treatment could be introduced at that stage, thus preventing the development of carcinoma of the cervix.

This test was introduced rapidly throughout the Western world, although in the absence of substantial evaluation. Subsequent evidence, particularly from Scandinavian countries, however, indicated that this was an effective screening test (Hakama, 1982). In Finland, Iceland and Sweden, for example, where a properly organized screening programme encompassing 80 percent of women between the ages of 25 and 60 years was introduced with regular rescreening, the incidence of invasive cervical cancer and consequent mortality rates from the condition were halved.

This has not been the experience in Britain as a whole where, despite many millions of cervical smears having been carried out over the last 20 years, there has been no change in mortality. The reason for this failure has been attributed to maldistribution of screening, with women at low risk having too frequent smears, whereas other women at high risk were not being screened at all. Nevertheless, in certain areas of Britain where screening programmes which reached most of the population, with rescreening at regular intervals, existed, the mortality rate has also been halved (Macgregor *et al.*, 1985). Day and his colleagues in 1986, reviewing the world literature, estimated that if all eligible women were screened every five years there would be a reduction in the incidence of invasive disease of 84 percent. Three-yearly screening would result in a 91 percent reduction (International Agency for Research in Cancer, 1986).

In Britain, women are usually invited for a cervical smear test by their primary care doctor, although there is increasingly the opportunity of attending a well women clinic. However, many women may be embarrassed by the thought of an internal examination and may be frightened by what the test may reveal. In addition, they may not believe that effective treatment is available if an abnormality is found. For the examiner, in contrast, cervical smear tests are straightforward and can be carried out relatively easily and quickly. Optimally, the woman should be notified of the result by post as soon as possible. Unfortunately, this has not always been the case. In the past women have often been led to believe "no news is good news", so that delays in communication have served to reassure, sometimes falsely, that there is no cause for concern. Current practice is both more sensitive and more stringent in this regard.

A number of women will be asked to attend for a repeat smear test for various reasons. The initial smear may have been unsatisfactory in that there were insufficient cells for a diagnosis to be made, or there may have been signs of infection or changes seen in the cells which could augur malignancy. The management of women in these latter circumstances has been the subject of some debate. While some have recommended that all women showing signs of cell abnormality be referred immediately for further examination and treatment, others contend that those showing only mild changes (known as mild dyskaryosis) should undergo a repeat smear within six months and, only if the abnormalities continue to be evident should there be an immediate referral.

Recently, the publication in the United Kingdom of *Guidelines for Clinical Practice and Programme Management NHS Screening Programme* (Duncan, 1992) has provided guidance on these matters. This guidance, drawn from available evidence, indicates that there is currently "no justification for managing mild dyskaryosis by immediate colposcopy" (p. 11). Rather, a smear should be repeated within six months and, only if the abnormality persists should further investigation take place.

Many people, including both providers and users of the service, have been concerned about the large numbers of women with mildly abnormal smears who have been referred each year for further examination and treatment. Williams, as part of a study to determine the type of information required for women diagnosed as having an abnormal cervical smear, interviewed a sample of 273 women referred for the first time to two colposcopy clinics in Glasgow. She summarized her findings as follows. "Women were very anxious about having an abnormal smear. In many cases, this anxiety was compounded by lack of information and professional support. The majority of women perceived themselves as very anxious, but also as coping well with the knowledge that they had an abnormal smear" (Williams, personal communication). The study reported that personal and social support systems were available for most women, who derived comfort and reassurance from them. Practical help was also valued. However, the knowledge status of some women was revealed as poor; they were ignorant of the purpose of cervical smears, the implication of an abnormal smear, or what treatment is involved. The main source of information was a leaflet sent out by the local clinic. Not all women made use of its contents and some apparently did not receive it. Most women indicated they would have benefitted from a video on the subject, or on audio tape. Discussion and information was important for many women; the desire for procedural, sensory, coping and reassuring information, was powerfully evident. Williams is currently designing an information and support package based on these findings, which will include a video with sign language and an audio tape for blind women and for those who have difficulty reading English (Williams, 1992).

Since 1988, in the UK, the National Screening Programme for cervical cancer has been operating and a system of regular computerized invitations for women aged 20–65 years registered with a general practitioner/primary care doctor has been in place. The aim of the programe is to reduce mortality from cervical cancer by screening all women at risk regularly in order to identify and treat conditions that otherwise might develop into cancer.

The program has specific goals which aim to ensure it is an efficient service, acceptable to women. These include efficient communication of results and appropriate treatment and follow-up, as well as effective monitoring of the programme. As such, the cervical screening programme has similar aims to the National Breast Screening Programme.

Screening for cancer of the breast

Breast cancer is the commonest form of cancer among British women. There are 22,000 new cases registered each year and 15,000 deaths from the condition. The UK mortality rate is higher than that recorded in the rest of Western Europe and North America (Forrest, 1986). The cause of the condition and means of prevention are as yet unknown. Accordingly, current evidence suggests the best way of reducing mortality is by screening women aged 50 years and over by X-ray mammography at regular intervals. No benefit has been demonstrated for screening of younger women. A major reason for this is that pre-menopausal breast tissue appears very dense on the mammogram making the detection of cancer difficult. Another problem is that breast cancer mortality rates are relatively low in women under the age of 50 and so research trials of young women frequently lack adequate statistical power. Additional trials of younger women are now in progress. As the best screening interval is not yet known, it is a subject of a large multicentre randomized controlled trial where three-yearly screening is being compared with an annual examination.

The organisation of the breast screening program in the UK is similar to that for cervical screening and is described in detail as it will help the reader to understand the various stages where problems may occur. The names of women in the relevant age group are obtained from the family doctors' lists of patients. A proposed list of women to be invited for screening is then drawn up. The family doctor vets this list to ensure that it is appropriate to invite all the women at this time. Occasionally there is an argument for postponing the invitation if, for instance, the women has experienced a recent bereavement. However, exclusions from invitation are rare; only women who have had a bilateral mastectomy or are terminally ill constitute *prima facie* exclusions.

A letter is then sent out inviting the women to come to a screening centre and an explanatory booklet is included along with instructions about how to reach the centre. A date and time are given, but it is explained clearly that, if the designated date is not convenient, an alternative will be arranged. The screening centres are in most cases outwith hospital settings, and are organized to appear as informal and unthreatening as possible. Every effort is made to reduce waiting to a minimum. Screening is then carried out and the woman is notified of the result as quickly as possible thereafter, ideally within one week of the test and certainly within two weeks. A survey of 3,000 women attending the 15 screening sites in Scotland during November, 1991, indicated that overall satisfaction with the program was high and that 88 percent of women confirmed they would return in three years' time. This was despite the fact that 53 percent of the women reported experiencing at least moderate discomfort during the examination and many women found the screening position uncomfortable (McIlwaine *et al.*, 1992). Ways of reducing the discomfort of the procedure are currently being investigated.

In approximately 10 percent of women, some abnormality was detected on the mammogram and a further test and clinical examination was therefore undertaken. Following this assessment, 15 percent of women (1.5 percent of those attending for initial screening) required further assessment by a surgeon; of these slightly less than half were revealed to have a cancer. In other words, for every 10,000 women screened, 1,000 will be recalled for a second examination, 150 will still have some abnormality on the second screen and around 65 women will actually have cancer of the breast. The randomized trials on which the UK programme was based reported a 30 percent reduction in mortality in the population invited for screening (Shapiro *et al.*, 1982; Taber *et al.*, 1985; Andersson *et al.*, 1988). This, of course, encompasses as a base those women who did not attend for screening. In the population who did attend, the reduction was actually 45 percent.

Similar studies were not undertaken when the cervical smear test was introduced, so comparisons between the two screening programmes are not possible.

FAILURE OF UPTAKE FOR CANCER SCREENING

It is obvious that if women do not attend for screening, the program will have no impact on mortality rates of the condition for which the screening program was introduced. It is therefore very important to uncover just what factors affect attendance.

Studies of cervical cancer screening programs reveal that women less likely to attend for screening are elderly, divorced or widowed and from lower socio-economic circumstances. The same has been found to be true for breast screening. The reasons given for non-attendance are often practical ones, such as family commitments, lack of time, problems with transport, etc. Hobbs and her colleagues (1985) pointed out that such reasons may indeed by true for many women. They also state, however, that under-representation of 'at risk' women has been attributed to the failure of the women to avail themselves of the screening facility. Such attributions are essentially victim-blaming and fail to take into account the characteristics of the service on offer. The responsiveness of the service to the needs of the women must be considered and Hobbs and her colleagues argue for a "provider-initiated, user-orientated system" (p. 262). Women must "know of the test's existence, have an understanding of its function and a belief both in its efficacy and its relevance to her" (p. 262). The nature of the experience of the test itself and its consequences must be acceptable.

Many of the difficulties outlined above should be minimized by the introduction of call/recall programs for both cervical and breast cancer screening. In such programes women are invited to attend and are provided with information about the test and how to obtain it. Every effort is made to make the service as user-friendly as possible. Nevertheless, even with such comparatively sensitive approaches, some women choose not to avail themselves of the service and so additional factors which affect non-attendance have therefore to be considered.

Data obtained from an Edinburgh breast screening study, which was set up in 1979 as a pilot project and forerunner of the national breast screening programme, are informative in this regard. French and colleagues (1982) compared a sample of attenders and non-attenders in their program, exploring whether the problem of non-attendance was one of administration or attitudes. The findings of the study suggest that non-attenders regarded a screening clinic as a place of risk, while the attenders harbored a more positive attitude. More than twice the numbers of non-attenders reported being frightened of cancer being discovered (79 percent versus 36 percent) and 72 percent of non-attenders, compared with only 13 percent of attenders, reported concern that their lives would be disrupted if cancer was found. A further study by MacLean *et al.* (1984) was undertaken, because of concern that low uptake (62 percent) could invalidate the outcome. The researchers found, in accord with other studies, that the non-attenders were from lower socioeconomic groups, made poor use of other preventative services, possessed limited knowledge of breast cancer and, in many cases, exhibited profound anxieties about the prospects of breast cancer screening. These researchers concluded that "both ethical and practical considerations oblige us to take serious note of what has come to light regarding women's views of the entire philosophy of screening for a symptomatic disease. Many women, it seems, do not automatically accept the value of such exercises" (p.280).

A subsequent Edinburgh study (Hunt *et al.*, 1988) also investigated factors related to attendance and non-attendance at the breast screening clinic. They concluded that explanation in terms of socio-economic characteristics alone was inadequate and oversimplistic. Non-attenders were revealed as a heterogeneous group with quite diverse reasons for not attending: some regarded screening as unnecessary; some harbored doubts about the efficacy of the test; others, because of the considerable strain imposed by their social circumstances were simply not in a position to consider screening.

Additional factors identified by Australian research as being positively related to attendance include: the intensity of thoughts about getting breast cancer; a belief that early detection is extremely desirable; a belief that screening mammograms are accurate; a belief that health is controlled by chance; and a feeling of personal susceptibility to breast cancer (Cockburn *et al.*, 1991).

Tymetra (1990) argued that in screening we are faced with the prevention-paradox, ie. "the benefit for some cannot be obtained without doing harm to others: many people undergo some stress, pain and anxiety in order to help others" (p. 60). In discussing why some people respond to an invitation for screening while others do not, Tymetra (1990) described a study in which women, who had recently given birth, were asked the hypothetic question "if screening tests (and adequate treatment) existed for a serious disease that occurred in only one in 90,000 babies would they be prepared to leave their baby in the screening centre for 24 hours so that those tests could be undertaken?" (p. 61). Thirty eight percent of respondents said they would and a further 29 percent wer eunsure. The author postulated that two factors, 'binary thinking' and 'anticipated decision regret', were important for over half of the subjects.

'Binary thinking' can be described as follows: when a new development offers the chance of a good outcome, some people do not consider the degree of risk, rather that a risk exists. It does not matter to that individual whether the risk is 1 in 100 or 1 in 10,000. In 'anticipated decision regret' the individual does not wish to blame herself for something going wrong. She will, therefore, decide to avail herself of every opportunity to ensure a good outcome. The individual might think "I do not want to blame myself later for not having tried everything I could" (Tymetra, 1990).

Other theories to be considered in relation to screening are the Health Belief Model (Becker *et al.*, 1977) and the Stress Coping Paradigm (Lazarus and Folkman, 1984). The Health Belief Model is explained simply by King (1984) as follows: "people are most likely to take preventive actions or to comply with professional medical advice if they feel concerned about their health and motivated to protect it; feel susceptible or at risk to the disease in question; believe that the consequences of the disease are serious if left untreated; believe in the recommended advice and treatment and that these outweigh any costs or drawbacks involved in following up this advice" (p. 54).

It would seem that this model might explain some of the differences found in attenders and non-attenders in the Edinburgh Breast Screening Programme. Calnan (1984) set up a study with the specific objective of examining the contribution the Health Belief model could make to explaining and predicting attendance at a screening clinic for X-ray mammography and attendance at a breast self-examination class. Analysis revealed that while health belief variables were among the best discriminators of take-up, the amount of variance in behavior explained by the variables in the Health Belief model was quite small and the predictive power of the model was generally low. A more recent study also used the Health Belief model to identify leading independent predictors of attendance at breast cancer screening (Fulton *et al.*, 1991). Among the predictors identified were recommendation by a medical provider, gynaecological care in the previous year, having a regular source of gynaecological care, having ever had a diagnostic mammogram, and perceiving mammography as safe enough to have annually.

In the social-psychological stress coping paradigm, the individual when confronted with a potential stressor has to pose and answer two questions: "What is the danger to me of the stressor?" and "What can I do about it?". The coping process is the manner in which the questions are answered and acted upon. Dealing with the first question is said to be primary appraisal. Assessing the threat and then determining what can be done following the primary appraisal, is said to be secondary appraisal (Folkman and Lazarus, 1984). It is obvious, therefore, that if the woman does not appraise herself to be at risk for the disorder to be screened for; or if she has no faith in the screening program to detect the disorder, or in the subsequent treatment, she will not avail herself of the service and will not attend.

The reasons why women do not attend for screening, therefore, are numerous, varied and complex, but all are important. The staff working in the screening service must be aware of these reasons and determine whether changes are required in the provision of their service in order to take into account the needs of women.

CONCLUDING REMARKS

Since the introduction of UK screening programs, particularly for breast screening, there have been a number of articles recording concern. The main areas of concern relate to the cost of these programs, the fact that they were introduced before publication of the pilot trials (which did not demonstrate clear efficacy) and the imperfect knowledge about the best way to treat breast cancer once it has developed.

Maureen Roberts, the clinical director of the Edinburgh Breast Screening program, died from breast cancer just as the British National Program was being introduced. She was concerned about many of the issues discussed above, and just before she died wrote an article for the *British Medical Journal* entitled "Breast cancer screening: Time for a rethink" (Roberts, 1989), in which she argues that "the Government is prepared to put a large amount of scarce resources into a national breast screening program, yet is unwilling to take on the tobacco industry at a political level, this despite overwhelming evidence that a truly preventive program would save thousands of lives each year from lung cancer and other diseases" (p.1155). Skrabanek (1989) posed another challenge, contending that "advocates of screening are more concerned with a cost-benefit analysis as it affects the whole population than with a harm-benefit analysis that affects the individual. They confuse statistical significance with practical relevance and benefits for society with benefits for the individual" (p. 428).

Where do we go from here? A National Breast Screening Program *has* been introduced. There is a highly organized quality control program in place and the service is being monitored very closely. Its preliminary findings are encouraging. Attendance has exceeded the 70 percent, predicted by the Forest Committee (1986), the recall rate is lower and the cancer detection rate higher than expected. It is essential, though, that the program continue for at least 10 years so that it be carefully monitored and evaluated (Vessey, 1991).

Two outstanding problems remain. How do we minimize anxiety in the five to ten percent of women recalled for further assessment who, on second examination are found not to have the disease? While some studies have apparently demonstrated a lack of long term anxiety, others have revealed that some women at least have higher rates of anxiety for up to a year after the screening, when compared with women who had not been recalled (Turnbull, 1992). More detailed population-based studies are currently underway measuring anxieties before invitation for screening, at the time of initial screen, at recall and three months and six months later (Cordiner, personal communication). A second area of concern is with subsequent rounds of screening. How do we maintain uptake or increase uptake where during the first round of screening it was low? Finally, in this context, it is important to address the question "What is meant by women's health?". In Britain, medical screening and family planning are regarded as almost synonymous with women's health within government and health service planning circles (McIlwaine, 1989). Wider issues of greater relevance to many women are simply not being addressed. In Australia, where a women's health policy has been adopted by the government, concern is much more broad-based encompassing: reproductive rights and sexuality; conditions associated with ageing such as osteoporosis, menopause, incontinence; mental health; violence against women; occupational health and safety; women as carers; sexual harassment (Special Consulate to the Minister for Commonwealth Department of Community Services and Health, 1988).

All these factors affect the health of many more women than the cancers that screening programmes aim to detect. It has been estimated, for instance, that 70 percent of women will consult their family practitioner at some time in their lives because of mental health problems. For half these women the problem will be recurrent. These other aspects of women's health must also be considered in the planning of health services for women and supported as generously as screening programs.

The Director General of the World Health Organization recognises that the issue of women's health goes even further. In his report Women, Health and Development (1985) he writes "women's health and roles depend on broad considerations – including employment, education and social status. Ultimately, they may even depend on equitable access to economic resources and political power. It is therefore imperative not to view the health aspects in isolation" (p. 1).

ACKNOWLEDGEMENTS

I would like to thank Deborah Turnbull for critical comments of an earlier draft and Carol Collins for typing the manuscript.

FURTHER READING

Forrest, P. (1986). *Breast cancer screening*. Report to the Health Ministers of England, Wales, Scotland and Northern Ireland. London: HMSO.
HMSO.
McIlwaine, G.M., Rowarth, M. and Wallace, A.M. (1992). Users views. Report of the Acceptibility Committee of the Scottish Breast Screening Service. Available on request to author.
Roberts, M.M. (1989). Breast screening: time for a rethink? *British Medical Journal*, **229**, 1153–1155.
Tymetra, T.J. (1990). Social and psychological repercussions of mass screening. In proceedings of the First World Congress "Safety in Medical Practice". Prevention and Compensation of Latrogenic Complications, Elisnore, Denmark, organised for ISPIC in collaboration with World Health Organisation Regional Office Europe, pp. 60–63.

11

CONTRACEPTION

ELIZABETH ALDER

Department of Management and Social Science, Queen Margaret College, Clerwood Terrace, Edinburgh EH12 8TS, UK

Despite the fact that overpopulation is a critical problem in many parts of the world, there has been relatively little research into the psychology of contraceptive use. Control over fertility has profound social implications, not least for women. Its importance for the psychology of women can hardly be overestimated, even though influential writers (eg. Ussher, 1989, Phoenix *et al.*, 1991) virtually ignore the topic. Specialist medical writers have largely neglected psychological aspects of contraception and even the relationship of contraception to sexual behavior has attracted little of their attention (eg. Guillebaud, 1991). Health psychologists have mainly addressed the problems of contraceptive choice in relation to adolescent use and as protection against AIDS, but there is much more than this to the psychology of contraception (Clarke, 1984).

This chapter will consider contraceptive choice; oral contraceptive pills and sterilization, reproductive strategies and the relationship of contraception to sexuality. Abortion is discussed in Chapter 3 and the use of condoms in Chapter 7.

CONTRACEPTIVE CHOICE

In the UK, under the 1972 National Health Service (Family Planning Amendment) Act, women are entitled to free contraceptive advice and supplies. These may be obtained from General (family) Practitioners or Family Planning Centres. Contraceptives can now also be bought over the counter from supermarkets and chemists, or from slot machines. Thus, few women are denied access to some kind of contraception in the UK, although the number of options may be limited in practice (Porter, 1991).

Contraceptive Use

Oral contraceptives are the first choice of contraception in the early years of reproductive life but there has been a fall in the popularity of oral contraceptives and a rise in the use of sheaths between 1976 and 1988 (Social Trends, 1990).

Population statistics can be baffling to psychologists interested in the behavior of the individual. There have been a number of significant events that have affected women's reproductive lives that may help to interpret the changes in contraceptive practice in the last 30 years. In the UK the Abortion Act, which increased access to abortion, took effect in 1968 and over the next decade contraception became more accessible through Government funded clinics and from family doctors from 1974 onwards. The oral contraceptive pill and IUD became available in the 1970's and in 1972 sterilization became free under the National Health Service. Hunt (1990) described contraceptive use in a cohort of over 800 UK men and women aged 35 in 1987/88. Eighty percent of these were using contraception; over 53 percent of whom had been sterilized (27 percent female and 26 percent male), 17 percent were using barrier methods, 13 percent used IUDs and 12 percent were using the oral contraceptive pill. When asked why they used a particular method of contraception they tended to give reasons in terms of the perceived disadvantages of the oral contraceptive pill rather than the advantages of other methods. Over 90 percent of this sample had used the pill at one time or another and 81 percent had used it as their first contraceptive method. Couples who are using contraception for the first time in the 1990's might well be influenced by the AIDS campaigns on condom use, but it is too early yet to tell what impact the spread of HIV infection might have on heterosexual contraceptive behavior.

Contraceptive Choice and Decision making

Women will have different demands and expectations of contraceptive methods at different times in their reproductive lives. The reproductive life cycle can be divided into three stages: sexually active before childbearing, childbearing with spaced pregnancies and the fertile years after childbearing is over. It is often assumed that reliability of contraception is more important in the first and last stages and that contraception should be matched to the appropriate stage. However, such assumptions are very much derived from a medical perspective of women and reproduction and may not take into account individual differences among women (Thomas, 1985).

Individual crises or points of transition may be more important than the sociocultural stage of child bearing and certainly more important than the exact chronological age. Changes in a relationship, a period of unemployment, ill health or a change in housing circumstances may all result in a change in the method of contraception. Side effects, dissatisfaction with the effect on sexual behavior, or a media scare may also prompt a change of method. However, most couples are fairly conservative in their choice. In a survey of 269 breast feeding women in 1986, it was found that most women used the same method before and after delivery of their first child (Alder, 1989).

The number of terminations and unplanned pregnancies remains high in spite of accessibility of contraception and not everyone uses contraception all of the time. Why should this be? There must be many couples who have taken a risk at some stage of their reproductive career. A belief in the safe period or in declining fertility, or being swept away by passion (or alcohol), or feeling unable to say 'no' may all accompany unprotected sexual intercourse. Pregnancy will follow few such occasions, but if it does the costs may be very high. There are strong pressures to use a safe and effective method of contraception but, as we shall see, contraceptive use is not without its costs.

It is relatively easy to obtain condoms, but obtaining other contraception may be regarded as a necessary, but not particularly pleasant medical errand rather like going to the dentist (Porter, 1991). The choice may then be influenced as much by the physician's preference as the woman's own cost/benefit analysis. Embarrassment or anxiety may also deter contraceptive use even at the point of obtaining supplies or advice from a health professional. Bruch and Haynes (1987) found that anxiety about heterosexual relationships correlated negatively with use of effective contraception at first intercourse. Research by social scientists concerned both with prevention of pregnancy and HIV/AIDS has concentrated on factors that influence contraceptive use during adolescence or pre-marital sexual activity. Large numbers of teenagers become pregnant each year, in spite of the free provision of contraceptives and sex education in schools. A number of models have been proposed to account for the use or non use of contraception by young people and the literature on premarital contraception has recently been reviewed (Scheeran *et al.*, 1991).

Models of Contraceptive Choice

The two predominant models of contraceptive decision-making are based on the concept of a contraceptive career or of a model of reasoned action or decision making. Lindemann (1977) described a 'contraceptive career' consisting of three stages. In the first 'natural stage', sexual intercourse is relatively rare and unplanned, and, since the woman does not perceive herself as a sexual being, she neither uses contraception nor takes responsibility for it. In the second 'peer prescription' stage there is more frequent sexual activity and a moderate acceptance of sexuality. At this stage she may seek information from intimate women friends but not from outside agencies. In the 'expert' stage she has incorporated sexuality into her self concept and so is more willing to use contraception that requires pre-planning and to seek contraceptive advice. There has been little direct empirical evaluation of the career model, although it does have some intuitive validity.

The decision model suggests that people weigh up the costs and benefits of the expected outcomes and the perceived probability of the outcomes. They then select the one that maximizes the benefits and minimizes the costs. If the expected benefits outweigh the expected costs then contraception will be used. Luker (1975) modeled the decision-making process. Risk taking is influenced by the subjective assessment of probability of pregnancy and the subjective assessment of the probability of obtaining an abortion. These operate with a costs/benefit balance of contraception and pregnancy and create an attitudinal set. Fishbein's model of reasoned action (Fishbein and Ajzen 1975) extends the subjective expected utility model to include both social influences and intention. Correlations of about 0.80 were found when the model was used to predict intention (Davidson and Jaccard, 1975) but actual behavior was not tested.

Whitely and Schofield (1986) considered contraceptive users and non users in a comprehensive meta analysis of 134 studies of adolescent contraception use. They found strong support for the career model for women but not for men. Sexual self acceptance was a major variable for both men and women supporting a central aspect of Linderman's career model. Other important variables were frequency of intercourse, age, self esteem and rejection of traditional sex roles. The decision model also received good support for women. The perceived risk of pregnancy (not surprisingly) was highly associated with contraceptive use. Positive attitudes to contraception and positive subjective norms were positively related to contraceptive use in women. The authors conclude that contraceptive use by young women is a function of the level of psychosexual maturity. A second factor is the decision-making process, which is constrained by the amount and quality of information that women possess (related to their career stage) and their perceived social norms. The third factor is the stage that a relationship has reached; contraception is more likely to be used if there is a stable sexual relationship.

Many models of lack of contraceptive use assume that the costs of non use outweigh the benefits and a number of studies have identified reasons for not using contraception or the disadvantages of using a particular method. These are most often *ex post facto*, recording justifications after the event rather than valid reasons for choice. Side effects have often been ignored in studies of contraceptive choice. In their review of 134 studies of adolescent contraceptive use, Whitely and Schofield (1986) did not include the cost of side effects as a variable in the testing of the decision making model.

CONTRACEPTIVE METHODS

The oral contraceptive pill has become the gold standard for pregnancy prevention, against which other methods may be compared. Its ease of use, reliability, relative lack of side effects and availability has undoubtedly raised the general expectations of contra-ceptive methods. Christopher (1991) claims that most women would prefer not to be bothered about contraception and the pill may be the least intrusive method. Sterilization may be the method of choice at the end of the reproductive career for the same reason. If the pill was the contraceptive phenomenon of the third quarter of the twentieth century, then sterilization will be so in the last quarter. These two methods will be considered in detail, although there are undoubtedly psychological implications of other methods, eg. the heavy menstrual bleeding of IUD's and interruption of sexual activity with barrier methods.

Oral Contraceptives

Oral contraceptives are of three main types: combined, sequential and progestagen only pills. Combined pills, which contain estrogen and progestogen, are taken for three weeks followed by a pill free week during which there is withdrawal bleeding. Sequential pills such as the tri-phasic pills give estrogen and progestogen for the first six days, followed by an increased dose of both for the next five days and then a high dose of progestogen for the last ten days accompanied by a lower dose of estrogen. A pill free week then follows. This pattern is thought to mimic the natural cycle. The progestogen only pills are taken continuously and there may be breakthrough bleeding. Recent prescriptions for combined and tri-phasic pills have included much lower doses of estrogen than the early preparations and this may make the results of early studies inapplicable to present day use.

Reduced sexual interest and depression were among the side effects reported by women taking these early oral contraceptives (Herzberg *et al.*, 1971). More recently, Warner and Bancroft (1988) analyzed the responses of over 4000 women to a questionnaire in a woman's magazine. They found that pill using women were more likely to report high sexual interest either during menstruation or during the preceding week and this was independent of their highs and lows of well being. Walker and Bancroft (1990) found that there was no difference in ratings of mood or sexuality in three groups of women on the triphasic pill, the combined pill or no pill, although the combined pill (monophasic) group reported less pre-menstrual breast tenderness than other groups. The results of studies of psychological effects of the pill may, however, be confounded by differences between women who are starting the pill and those who have used it for a number of years. Those who experience side effects drop out, leaving those without side effects to become long term users. They are more likely to have tried a number of different preparations until they have found one that suits them. There may also be a period of adjustment to a new hormonal regime and the pattern of withdrawal bleeding often settles down after a few months. Some women may also be more disposed to cyclical changes and these may be augmented or suppressed by the use of oral contraceptives. This is a very complex area and one in which research is badly needed.

The benefits of the oral contraceptive pill are far reaching, but physical side effects do occur and the use of contraception is not without risk, whatever the method. High dose estrogen oral contraceptives have been associated with increased risk of thromboembolic disorders, stroke and heart disease, although the risks are much reduced in low dose or progestagen only pills (Population Reports, 1988). The concept of risk derived from epidemiological studies is difficult to interpret and risks are not always put into context. The risk of death per 100,000 people is 1.3 for non smoking pill users whereas it is 17 per 100,000 for average mileage car drivers (Guillebaud, 1991a). Combined oral contraceptives usually induce a decrease in menstrual flow that may be very welcome, but some progestagen only pills may cause break-through bleeding. Menstrual disturbances such as break-through bleeding may not be tolerated. The unpredictability of menstrual bleeding may cause anxiety about 'normality' in women as well as being simply inconvenient (Fraser 1986). If a method of contraception has adverse effects, many users will change their method. It is very easy to give up oral contraceptives.

The considerable influence of the media on oral contraceptive use was shown by the pill scare of 1983. Two papers published in the *Lancet* in October 1983 suggested a link between contraceptive pill use and cancer (Pike *et al.*, 1983, Vessey *et al.*, 1983) and the number of prescriptions for oral contraceptives in England and Wales dropped by 14 percent in the following month (Wellings, 1985). The dramatic effects of this pill scare suggest that not only are women vigilant in their search for information but that their long term health has high priority. This will be no surprise to many psychologists or to women themselves. However, reference to 'don't panic' in the newspaper headlines suggested that journalists did not view contraceptive choice by women as being based on a rational decision-making model. Women may thus be stereotyped as being ignorant or emotional. The medical profession may also be anxious about women taking over control of their contraceptive method.

Oral contraceptive pills are commonly regarded as being reliable and easy to use, yet missing a pill is an important cause of unplanned pregnancy (Metson, 1988). Brook and

Smith (1991) surveyed 40 pill users and found that only half knew that missing a pill, diarrhoea/vomiting or taking antibiotics might reduce their protection, and 40 percent did not know which brand of oral contraception they were taking. If one combined pill is missed by more than 12 hours, women are advised that the missing pill should be taken and additional contraception used for at least 14 days. In a study of 200 women taking the combined pill (Metson *et al.*, 1991), half were given verbal instruction (control group) and half were given an instruction leaflet (leaflet group). One year later the subjects were asked what they would do if they missed a pill. Only 18 (20 percent) of the leaflet group and only 3 (2 percent) of the control group knew what to do. Thus, knowledge of what to do if the pill was missed was greater in the leaflet group, but still strikingly low. We know that compliance with medication is generally poor (Ley, 1988) but we might expect that it would be higher if a pregnancy could result from non compliance. Improving compliance rates has been a fruitful area of health psychology research and Ley (1988) gives a comprehensive and readable account of relevant issues.

Ovarian activity is more likely to follow if an oral contraceptive pill is forgotten at the beginning of a packet (at the end of a pill free week) than one forgotten in mid cycle. The style of packaging can reduce the risk of forgetting by including seven dummy pills for the 'pill free' week. This makes taking the pill a regular daily practice. Of course, taking a contraceptive pill may be influenced by more subtle psychological factors than those involved in taking for example, antibiotics, and consequently one argument against the use of a male pill is that women may doubt that men could be trusted to take it regularly (Guillebaud, 1991a). The assumption must be that several million men trust women to take the present oral contraceptive pill! This surely tells us something about differences in the relative costs of pregnancy to men and women including the perceived and actual responsibilities for child rearing.

Sterilization

The most prevalent birth control method world-wide is voluntary female sterilization. In November 1990 it was estimated that 138 million women were protected from unwanted pregnancy by voluntary female sterilization, representing about 16 percent of all married women of reproductive age (Population Reports, 1990). In developed countries it is particularly popular. The number of women relying on sterilization to prevent pregnancy in the US rose from 17 percent in 1982 to 23 percent in 1988. There are differences even within developed countries eg. only 6 percent of women are sterilized in Sweden and in Rumania sterilization only became legal in 1990 (Population Reports, 1990). Laparoscopic sterilization became widely used in the 1970's and became popular because it was a simple and effective surgical procedure, involved only one post operative check, no provision of supplies, few side effects and had a low failure rate. From the woman's point of view the operation may be attractive because it can be done on a day care basis, leaves only two small scars and is safe. However, sterilization operations are effectively irreversible and it is very difficult to repair fallopian tubes successfully, although there is a chance of conception using in vitro fertilization (IVF) which could lead to sterilization being regarded as a temporary contraceptive method (Dawson and Singer, 1990). Nevertheless, conception rates with IVF are low and both partners suffer emotional stress (Chan *et al.*, 1989). Limited access and financial costs mean that it is unlikely to be a realistic option for many couples.

Follow up studies of women after sterilization have generally reported favorable results. In a retrospective study of over 500 patients only 2 percent complained about physical problems (Lawson *et al.*, 1979). Women who have been sterilized who had previously been on the pill may have more menstrual problems once they return to normal menstrual cycles. Alder *et al.*, (1981) found that women who had been sterilized reported more menstrual changes both positive and negative, compared with the wives of vasectomized men. There is always concern that a woman may later regret her decision to be sterilized and regret rates obtained from prospective studies vary from 2 to 10 percent. The early follow up studies of sterilization reviewed by Schwyhart and Kutner (1973) found regret rates of between 3 and 15 percent, but later prospective studies reported lower rates (eg. Cooper *et al.*, 1982). Lambers *et al.*, (1984) identified the factors associated with regret following sterilization as being: lack of freedom of choice in the decision-making process; a belief that the sterilization operation would solve other problems; an inability to cope with loss of fertility; and a strong adherence to a sex role identity that was linked to reproductive capacity. However, many studies in this area suffer from methodological flaws such as having low response rates, no control groups, potential interviewer bias, or being retrospective, (Lambers *et al.*, 1984). Nevertheless, most researchers conclude that there is a need for counseling before the decision is made.

At one time there was a guiding rule that parity multiplied by age should be equal to 120 or more before women should be considered for sterilization. This no longer applies in practice, although many doctors would be reluctant to carry out sterilization of either men or women in their early twenties. There is some evidence for more regret if women are sterilized at a young age. There is also an increased risk of marital breakdown in those who marry young and some women who regret the operation and ask for a reversal want to have children in a new relationship. In a study of 34 women requesting reversal of sterilization in New Zealand, 30 were in a new marital relationship and 23 of them believed that they had been suffering from significant anxiety or depression at the time that they had been sterilized (Romans-Clarkson and Gillett, 1987). In our retrospective study six women expressed some regret. These consisted of two whose housing conditions had improved, one whose marriage had broken down, one because of a perceived loss of femininity, one who wanted more children and one because of menstrual problems that began after she had stopped taking the oral contraceptive pill (Alder *et al.*, 1981).

REPRODUCTIVE STRATEGIES

Family planning has come to mean the provision of contraceptive advice, but choosing an optimal reproductive strategy may also be a source of concern to many women. The timing of the first child, spacing of births, the number of children and the gender balance may all influence reproductive strategies and hence contraceptive choice.

Most Western studies find that very few married couples prefer to remain childless, but it has been argued that in the UK and the US there is a pronatalist culture where parenthood is seen as the legitimate goal of most married couples (Campbell, 1985). The financial costs and the physical and emotional costs of childbearing have been well documented. The choice of contraceptive method for the voluntary childless (or childfree) may be more strongly influenced by reliability than other factors. Sterilization is an obvious choice at the point where the commitment to voluntary childlessness is total.

Woollett *et al.*, (1991) in a study of Asian women living in London found that most women expected to become mothers. Some wanted to have their first child soon after marriage and to have a second child soon after the first. These women tended not to have used contraception before the birth of the first child and were interested in limiting family size only when they had two or three children. Others wanted to delay the birth of the first child for two or three years until their marriages or finances were well established. Half of the 32 women interviewed had given birth within 15 months of marriage. The women balanced the benefits of spending only a few years caring for young children by having them close together, against reducing the effort by having them more widely spaced out.

Cartwright (1987) compared trends in contraceptive use of women in the UK between 1976 and 1984. The percentage of mothers with one child who said that they hoped to have more children fell from 85 percent in 1967 to 75 percent in 1984. There has also been a trend to later motherhood despite the concept of the 'right' time to have children and prejudice against older mothers (Berryman, 1991). The increase in the use of permanent methods of contraception involving sterilization has undoubtedly reduced family size in the last few decades. Guillebaud (1991b) suggests that women are more motivated towards family planning just after childbirth than at any other time but that they may also be vulnerable to pressures from the medical profession. Women who have been sterilized after delivery are at greater risk of regretting the operation and sterilization is consequently often delayed for three to six months. The oral contraceptive pill is the most frequently used method during child bearing years and there has been little change in the last 15 years. The use of the pill decreased with increasing family size. It is now an accepted part of Western culture, at least in non Catholic countries, that the number of children is a matter for choice. In a recent survey of about 400 35-year old women, those who chose sterilization had previously used effective methods, such as the oral contraceptive pill for longer (Hunt and Allendale, 1990). The authors suggest that increased expectations of contraceptive efficacy have contributed to the recent rise in popularity of sterilization. Whether the woman considered her family complete was a much more important determinant of choice of contraceptive method than any of the socio-economic, health, or other reproductive variables. Sterilization operations are now taking place at a younger age and at lower levels of parity, suggesting that the reproductive strategy of the future is to limit family size and make this effectively an irreversible decision.

CONTRACEPTION AND SEXUALITY

It is difficult to demonstrate a consistent effect of contraception on sexual behavior. Women who take the pill are more sexually active than those using other methods or none at all (Westoff *et al.*, 1976), but women who choose to use oral contraception may do so because of their level of sexual activity. There could also be endocrine mediated effects on sexual behavior in pill takers, although these have been difficult to demonstrate. Attribution of sexual problems to hormonal changes is common and the expectations of first time pill users may differ from those who have been using it for some time. Olasov and Jackson (1987) demonstrated the effect of expectation of negative change on mood and health. Goetsch *et al.*, (1991) found in a study of 19 first time users in a contraceptive education programme, that 13 (65 percent) expected at least one negative effect. The possibility of an adverse effect of sterilization on sexual relationships has been considered in a number of studies (see discussion by Alder, 1984b; Hunter, 1989), but the results have been conflicting. Wright (1978) found that 28 percent of sterilized women had sexual problems compared with 13 percent of non sterilized women in a postal questionnaire, but Bean *et al.* (1982) found that 25 percent of sterilized women reported an increase in sexual desire 6 months after the operation. In our interview study we found that 7 percent of sterilized women reported a deterioration of sexual relationships although none of the wives of vasectomized men thought that their relationship had worsened (Alder *et al.*, 1981). The differences could reflect the effect of the operations or the differences between couples seeking male or female sterilization. They could also reflect the counseling that was given to the couples seeking male vasectomy but not female sterilization. This opportunity for discussion may have also helped their sexual relationship. In looking at the consequences of contraception it is important to remember that a particular contraceptive method may be chosen *because* of the nature of the sexual relationship.

Given that sterilization is non intrusive and allows spontaneous and uninterrupted sexual activity, it seems surprising that it was initially associated with adverse effects on sexual relationships. A diagnosis of male infertility frequently alters sexual relationships (Alder, 1984a) and sterilization effectively makes one partner sterile. It is this association of sexuality with fertility that has caused anxieties about permanent methods of contraception. Thus, for some couples sex without any risk of pregnancy may be less exciting. This possibility is at odds with the rational analysis of contraceptive decision-making presented earlier, but some couples report that sexual intercourse has an added meaning when no contraception is used. Intuitively it seems that having sex *in order* to conceive may differ from sex where there is *some risk* of conception and differs again from sex when there is *no possibility* of conception.

Pregnancy may be the only time during the reproductive career that the couple feel completely free from concerns about contraception or conception and sex can be uninhibited and spontaneous. However, the frequency of sexual activity declines as pregnancy progresses and for most women there is also a decline in satisfaction. Towards the end of pregnancy the couple may be eagerly awaiting the birth of their child but they may also look forward to renewing their sexual relationship. There is evidence from a number of studies that there is a very low return to previous levels of sexual activity and satisfaction. Masters and Johnson (1966) suggested that most couples resumed sexual intercourse by six to eight weeks following delivery but later studies that were prospective and had larger samples showed a slower return, although there was considerable individual variation. Factors contributing to this slow return include changes in body image, fatigue, breast feeding, hormonal changes and fear of pregnancy (Alder, 1989).

Surprisingly, few studies of sexual behavior in the puerperium asked about contraception (eg. Reamy and White; 1987). Guillebaud (1991b) suggests that contraceptive counseling should be given antenatally, although experience of parent craft classes shows that prospective parents are often reluctant to discuss anything other than the delivery. Ovulation can occur as early as day 30 following delivery in non lactating mothers but is much later and more variable if the woman is fully breast feeding. Following delivery the combined oral contraceptive pill may be unsuitable because of its effect on lactation. Mothers using combined oral con-traceptives have a shorter lactation period, but no adverse effects on the baby's growth or psychological development have been shown (Nilsson *et al*, 1986). If they missed a pill or stopped taking it all together they would be at risk of pregnancy earlier. Lactation has a contraceptive effect because of the effect on the endocrine mechanism but it may also influence sexual behavior (Sudlow, 1991).

If the mother is fully breast feeding almost all methods of contraception will be effective but some may carry a slight risk of affecting the breast milk. The progestagen pill is the method most often suggested to lactating mothers, but even so some women may have doubts about taking hormones and prefer to use barrier methods. There is a dilemma here, the chances of conception are low but another pregnancy soon after the first may have very high physical, financial and emotional costs. Although sexual intercourse may be infrequent, the couple may wish it to be spontaneous and may even compare it to the early days of worry free pregnancy. Their reproductive strategy and their own sexual activity will affect their choice of contraceptive method during the childbearing years.

CONTRACEPTION AND HEALTH

There is no doubt that reduction in family size has improved the physical health of women. The life expectancy has risen dramatically over the last 100 years in the UK. It is also rising in the developing countries where the average parity is falling (Social Trends, 1990). The ability of women to control their fertility frees them from the physical burden of repeated pregnancies and caring for children but it also gives them freedom from dependence on men as providers. It can be no coincidence that in Western countries effective contraception has been accompanied by increasing female employment outside the home.

Self efficacy is the belief in the ability to accomplish things and that one is not at the mercy of forces beyond one's control (Bandura, 1977). An effective method of contraception should increase this sense of self efficacy and therefore help women to cope with other stressful events. The research on decision control (Taylor, 1986) emphasizes the importance to women of making their own decisions about contraceptive choice.

ISSUES

Most women are likely to be affected by their choice of contraception at some point in their lives. The relationship between contraceptive choice and the desire to avoid pregnancy is not a straightforward one and inevitably involves aspects of the couple's sexual relationship. This might suggest that basic research into understanding the psychology of contraceptive use is essential, before new physical or pharmacological methods are developed.

The AIDS campaign has increased public awareness of sexual activity among young people and yet an over emphasis on the use of condoms, which are far from reliable contraceptives, may increase the risk of unwanted pregnancy. The issue is whether women will bother to take the oral contraceptive pill as well as insisting on condoms.

The question of responsibility for contraception is still debated and the role of the male partner, perhaps underemphasized during the hey-day of the oral contraceptive pill, is likely to receive more attention in future. The development of a male pill may not be too far away but will women trust men to take it?

In the developing world lactation is an important factor in limiting births. This raises the question of whether more effort should be spent promoting breast feeding (which would entail curbing the activities of multinational dried milk companies) rather than supplying contraceptives.

Complex questions are always raised when we consider the psychology of reproduction but psychologists should surely make more attempt to answer them when so many questions are asked by so many people.

Acknowledgements

I would like to thank Sally Wyke and Anne Walker for their helpful comments on this chapter.

FURTHER READING

Alder, E. (1989). Sexual behaviour in pregnancy, after childbirth and during breastfeeding. In M.R. Oates (Ed.), *Psychological aspects of obstetrics and gynaecology, Bailliere's clinical obstetrics and gynaecology 3, no 4*. London: Bailliere Tindall.

Royle, M. (1991). Decision making for contraception and abortion. In M. Pitts and K. Phillips (Eds.), *The Psychology of health: An introduction*. London: Routledge.

Hunt, K. (1990). The first pill taking generation: past and present use of contraception among a cohort of women born in the early 50's. *The British Journal of Family Planning*, 9, 3–15.

Scheeran, P., White, D. and Phillips, K. (1991). Premarital contraceptive use: a review of the psychological literature. *Journal of Reproductive and Infant Psychology*, 9, 253–269.

12

GENDER, SOCIAL CIRCUMSTANCES AND HEALTH

DOUGLAS CARROLL, CATHERINE A. NIVEN AND DAVID SHEFFIELD

Department of Psychology, Glasgow Polytechnic, Cowcaddens Road, Glasgow G4 0BA, UK

In the opening chapter of this text, we alluded to the links between health and social and material circumstances. Whether indexed by occupational status or by asset-based measures such as household income (Blaxter, 1990) or housing tenure and car ownership (Whitehead, 1988), those at the top of the social scale enjoy substantially lower rates of mortality than those further down. The mortality differentials contingent on social locus typify women as much as they do men (see, eg. Whitehead, 1988). Further, what is true of mortality also applies to morbidity. All the major killer disease groups now affect the less well off more than the rich (Davey Smith *et al.*, 1990). Long-standing illness measures also favour higher income groups (see, eg. Arber, 1989; Blaxter, 1989). Again these morbidity differentials characterize women as much as men (see, eg. Marmot *et al.*, 1991). What seems to be emerging from recent epidemiological research then, is a gradient of morbidity and mortality that applies to both men and women and persists throughout the social and occupational scale. Accordingly, the implications of social and material circumstances for health appear to extend beyond the very poor in society.

While variations in mortality and morbidity with social and material circumstances seem to be characteristic of all Western countries (see, eg. Fox, 1989), the magnitude of the differential differs among countries. There has now been, at least as far as mortality is concerned, some preliminary exploration of the possible sources of such variation. Evidence is emerging that income distribution may be the key.

Wilkinson (1990, 1992) compared data on income distribution and life expectancy for nine Western countries (Australia, UK, Canada, Netherlands, Norway, Sweden, Switzerland, US, West Germany). Whereas Gross National Product was not associated with life expectancy at birth, income distribution (defined as the percentage

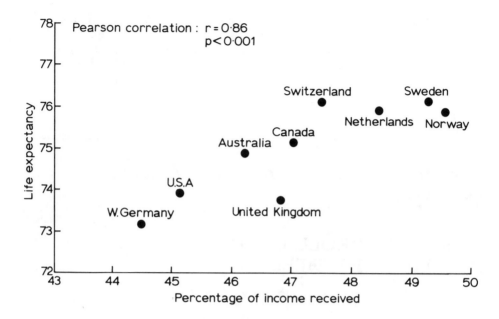

FIGURE 12.1   Relationship between life expectancy at birth (male and female combined) and percentage of post tax and benefit income received by the least well off 70 percent of families, 1981. (Adapted from Wilkinson, 1992 and reproduced by permission of the British Medical Journal).

of a country's total post-tax income and benefit received by the least well-off 70 percent of 'families') yielded a substantial positive correlation ($r = 0.86$). Figure 12.1 presents these data. It is interesting to note that this analysis did not include Japan. The Japanese now have the longest life expectancy in the world (Marmot and Davey Smith, 1989) and also the most equitable distribution of income of any Organization for Economic Cooperation and Development country (Wilkinson, 1992). Subsequent analyses of 12 European Community countries by Wilkinson (1992) indicate that for the years 1975–85, the annual rate of change in life expectancy was negatively correlated with another measure of income distribution: in this case, the proportion of the population in relative poverty, defined as those living on less than 50 percent of the national average disposable income. Again, the correlation coefficient was substantial ($r = -0.73$), indicating that a more rapid improvement in life expectancy was enjoyed by those countries which had registered a fall in the prevalence of relative poverty. What emerges from these analyses is that life expectancy relates not just to how wealthy countries are but how that wealth is distributed.

Thus, for most people in Western countries, health hinges on relative rather than absolute living standards. This implies that it is the psychosocial parameters of people's lives rather than the physical fabric *per se* that primarily affect health. As Wilkinson (1992) concluded "It looks as if what matters about our physical circumstances is not what they are in themselves, but where they stand in the scale of things in our society. The implication is that our environment and standard of living no longer impact on our health primarily through direct physical courses, regardless of our attitudes and perceptions, but have come to do so mainly through social and cognitively mediated processes (p. 405). What might these psychosocial parameters be? Wilkinson (1992) speculates that gross social and material division might have widely distributed effects on, among other things, the quality of social relations and the quantity of psychosocial stress. We have already examined the role of the latter in the opening chapter. For the rest of this chapter let us turn our attention to the former and, in particular, to the possible implications of aspects of social relations for gender differences in health.

SOCIAL SUPPORT

Much of the research on social relations and health has been carried out under the rubric of social support, which may be briefly defined as the comfort, caring, esteem, or help provided by other people or social groups. However, this rather simple definition conceals considerable complexity. For example, as Cohen and Syme (1985) pointed out, social support processes have been studied from two somewhat different perspectives. In some cases support has been conceptualized mainly in terms of the structure of relations (eg. number of relationships, their intimacy); elsewhere, the focus has been on the functions that relationships or social networks serve (eg. emotional support, material assistance). As those latter examples indicate, social support can fulfil both affective and instrumental functions, providing for a sense of belonging, of being loved and needed in the former and for practical assistance, financial, physical, or material, in the latter (Miles, 1991). Moreover, measures of 'social support' may reflect negative aspects of an individual's social interactions. Consider for instance the person who has a large social network defined as people s/he interacts with on a regular basis. You might think of a student sharing a residence with a substantial number of fellow students. The interactions between these individuals may be negative rather than positive and may be characterized by social destruction rather than support. Similarly, parents may continue to provide material assistance in the form of financial support to their offspring while they are at college or university, or are unemployed. Although this assistance can be welcome, it may be a source of resentment for both parents and young adults and thus may make it less likely that mutual caring, esteem and emotional support are available. Given such complexities and the variety of operational definitions of social support employed by researchers, it is hardly surprising that there are some inconsistencies in outcome. Nevertheless, a number of recurring messages emerge from the various investigations into social support and health; individuals evidencing relatively low levels of social support would seem to suffer from increased mortality from a range of causes, increased morbidity and poor prognoses and retarded recovery in a number of contexts.

SOCIAL SUPPORT AND HEALTH

A number of prospective studies have been reported and all confirm that in general those exhibiting the lowest levels of social support suffer the highest rates of morbidity. For example, Berkman and Syme (1979) reported that mortality over a nine-year period was linearly related to a social network index which measured the extent of individuals' family, social and community ties: those with fewest ties suffered the highest rates of mortality. The effect held for both men and women and was evident for specific causes of death, such as ischaemic heart disease and cancer, as well as for overall all-cause mortality. House *et al.* (1982) also found that all-cause mortality over a 10-year period was related to social support, assessed in much the same way as the previous study. However, the effect was significant for men only and was non-linear, ie. while very low levels of social support disadvantaged men, subsequent increases in social support above the middle range yielded no further benefit. Schoenbach *et al.* (1986) again interviewed participants at the outset about their family, social and community relationships and tracked mortality for a subsequent 11 years. For the older age group, ie. men and women over 60, low social support was associated with increased mortality. Again, the relationship was nonlinear, most of the effect being accounted for by the lowest level of social support. In contrast, though, for women under 60, higher social support scores were associated with higher mortality rates.

By far the largest study to date, encompassing over 17000 Swedish men and women was conducted by Orth-Gomer and Johnson (1987). Participants were interviewed at the outset concerning their social network and interactions and a composite score derived to characterize the extent of their social contact. Mortality was examined during a six year follow-up period during which 841 of the participants had died. Dividing social support scores into high, medium and low, it was observed that mortality rates for both men and women under 65 years old were highest for those with the lowest support scores; there were no differences in mortality between those with medium and those with high support scores. Similar effects emerged for cardiovascular disease-specific mortality rates. However, the results for older participants were more complex. For men, there was a linear relationship between the measure of social contact and mortality; for older women, though, high social support was associated with increased mortality.

Overall, these studies consistently affirm that men appear to benefit from enhanced social support, although there does seem to be a threshold effect, such that low levels of support disadvantage, but support beyond moderate levels adds little additional benefit. The picture for women, however, is far less clear.

Turning now to morbidity, prognosis and recovery, the volume and quality of evidence is less persuasive, but does seem to point in the same general direction. In a study of coronary artery disease, Blumenthal *et al.* (1987) reported an interaction between social support and type A behavior, such that individuals manifesting type A behaviour but with high levels of social support displayed lower levels of coronary artery disease than type A individuals with low levels of social support. In general, the Blumenthal group have found that type A behavior is associated with the presence of coronary artery disease (see, eg. Bennett and Carroll, 1990, for a review). However, the present study included few women and no gender-specific analyses were reported. There is at least preliminary evidence that social support may reduce pregnancy complications, at least for women exposed to recent life stresses (see, Berkman, 1985). For example, Norbeck and Tilden (1983) found higher incidences of gestation complications and infant condition complications in women registering many life stresses and low levels of social support. Formal provision of social support by midwives to pregnant women at risk of having a low birthweight baby has also been found to be associated with significantly improved fetal, infant and maternal outcomes (Oakley *et al.*, 1990). However, the overall pregnancy picture is complex. For example, in terms of labor and delivery complications it was low social support in association with few life stresses in the Norbeck and Tilden study that yielded the highest incidence. The provision of social support during childbirth by the laboring woman's chosen birth companion has been found in some studies to be associated with lower levels of labor pain (Niven, 1985) when the companion's presence was welcome, but in others the presence of the parturant's husband was associated with higher levels of reported pain (Melzack, 1984). Klaus, Kennel and colleagues (1986) have reported reduced rates of complications where women in childbirth have been accompanied by a *doula* – a lay women who gave constant emotional and physical support during labor and delivery. In the most recent of their studies which were carried out in a modern US hospital, a doula-accompanied woman had significantly lower rates of epidural anaesthesia, forceps assisted deliveries, and Caesarean sections compared with a control group. Social support factors have been implicated in both the development and alleviation of post-natal depression. For instance, Elliot *et al.* (1988) have found that lack of emotional support and a confiding relationship as well as a poor marital relationship are associated with post-natal depression. They subsequently developed a perinatal prevention program which placed a major emphasis on the formal and informal provision of social support for women at risk of post-natal depression and which was successful in significantly reducing the incidence of post-natal depression in mothers having their first baby. However, factors other than social support are involved in the development and resolution of post-natal depression and the concept of *post-natal* depression itself continues to be a source of debate. Finally, there is some evidence that social support has implications for disease prognosis. Funch and Marshall (1983), for example, found that among women with breast cancer, those with higher levels of social involvement enjoyed significantly longer survival. More recently, Fontana *et al.*, (1989) studied a group of men who had been admitted to hospital following myocardial infarction or had undergone bypass surgery. They were followed up for 12 months after discharge and various measures of stress, social support and cardiac symptomatology taken. Psychological stress was found to exacerbate cardiac symptomatology, while social support ameliorated the subsequent experience of stress and had the opposite effects to stress on cardiac symptomatology.

Two questions immediately arise. What mechanisms might underly these social support effects? Why, at least in terms of the mortality studies, does social support appear to afford less of a protection for women than for men?

MECHANISMS OF SOCIAL SUPPORT

Schumaker and Hill (1991) posited several possible mechanisms. First of all, social support might work by promoting healthy behaviors. There is some evidence, for example, that social support increases adherence to medical advice. In a study of hypertensive men Doherty *et al.* (1983) asked wives about their beliefs and behaviors possibly relevant to their husbands' antihypertensive medication. Adherence was reliably better in men with supportive wives who believed in the benefits of the treatment. However, it was positive support, interest and encouragement that proved effective. Doherty *et al.* found that where wives nagged their husbands about medication, adherence was relatively poor. In addition, as Cohen and Syme (1985) suggested, the perception that others are willing to help could result in increased senses of self-esteem, stability and control over the environment, which, in turn, may reduce the likelihood of recourse to unhealthy substances such as tobacco and alcohol and change the value attached to diet and exercise. However, we are without much direct evidence of such effects. Recently, though, Dean (1989) presented evidence that self-reported health care behavior was positively related to social support, although the effects were more evident for men than for women. Men with larger friendship networks more often reported behavioral practices to maintain health. Instrumental support from the network was associated with regular physical activity in men and available extended family with reduced male alcohol consumption.

Secondly, it has been argued that social support may yield dividends through more tangible means by, for example, the provision of economic aid. There is certainly preliminary evidence that benefits can accrue from economic assistance to the materially disadvantaged. Kehrer and Wolin (1979) reported a study in Gary, Indiana, of the effects of income supplementation through negative income tax on birthweight. Compared to low income mothers who had not received benefit, the risk of low birthweight babies was significantly reduced for mothers in poor families who were receiving income supplement. A French initiative based in Alsace used income supplementation to compensate pregnant women financially for absence from employment which entailed heavy physical work. This reduced the incidence of very low birthweight in women at medium risk (Papiernik *et al.*, 1985). However, the researchers also provided some of the subjects with a 'family worker' who provided social and practical support and increased obstetric monitoring and domiciliary midwife visiting. Thus, a number of factors as well as income supplementation may have affected the results. Direct nutritional supplementation through the provision of food vouchers along with nutritional education in a Massachusetts study significantly reduced low birth weight and nutritional mortality of participant women compared with matched controls (Kotelchuck *et al.*, 1984).

Thirdly, the positive psychological states that derive from social support may buffer the physiological impact of psychological stress, either directly or by altering the appraisal of stressful events. A number of recent studies have examined this issue. Kamark *et al.* (1990) monitored the cardiovascular reactions of college-age women to two laboratory stressors in two situations: alone, or accompanied by a friend, instructed to act as a non-evaluative supporter, remaining silent but touching the subject on the wrist. In the latter context, women showed reduced heart rate and systolic blood pressure reactions to stress, although in the case of systolic blood pressure the effect was statistically significant for only one of two laboratory stress tasks. This result, however, is very much at odds with the findings of Allen *et al.* (1991). Forty-five women performed a mental arithmetic stress task in the laboratory with only the experimenter present, during which time physiological activity was measured. Two weeks later, measurements were repeated at the subjects' homes, again during mental arithmetic challenge. In the home condition, however, subjects were tested either alone, in the presence of a pet dog, or with a female friend present. In contrast to the previous study, subjects in the friend condition exhibited more marked heart rate, systolic blood pressure and skin conductance reactions to stress than subjects in the other two conditions. Attenuation of these physiological reactions was evident only in the pet dog condition. Allen *et al.* interpreted their results in terms of the degree to which friends and pet dogs are regarded as evaluative. Evaluative appraisals, it was conjectured, would serve to increase stress and consequent physiological reactivity. In Kamark *et al.*'s study, the protocol was designed to optimize subjects' appraisals of partners as non-evaluative and supportive. In a subsequent study, Edens *et al.* (1992)

found that the presence of a friend did reduce the physiological impact of psychological stress; female subjects tested with a friend displayed smaller reactions than females tested with a stranger. Clearly, there is much to resolve here; the precise demeanour of the partner in the circumstances of stress exposure would appear to be crucial, as would the closeness of the relationship between subject and partner. Illustration of this emerges from a recent study by Spitzer *et al.* (1992). Ambulatory blood pressure levels were monitored every 20 minutes for a 12-hour period in 131 normotensive or mildly hypertensive men and women. Blood pressure varied significantly as a function of the social situation (alone, with family, with friends or with strangers). Blood pressure levels were lowest when subjects were with family and highest when subjects were with strangers.

Many of the effects of social support on pregnancy outcome are assumed to be related to the effects of offsetting stress on the mother and consequently on the fetus, (see eg. Newton, 1988). Stress in pregnant animals was observed to be followed by a rise in maternal noradrenaline (norepinephrine) and a fall in uterine blood flow (Levinson and Schnider, 1979). Bontekoe and colleagues (1977) found that the effect of maternal stress on uterine muscle contractibility was dependent on plasma sex steroid concentrations. In early or mid pregnancy maternal stress may increase uterine muscle contractibility causing miscarriage or premature labor, whereas in late pregnancy when estrogen predominates it may inhibit contractibility, thus prolonging labor. In humans, Lederman *et al.* (1978) demonstrated that during labor, mothers' reports of anxiety were correlated with higher levels of maternal adrenaline (epinephrine), lower levels of uterine contractibility and longer duration of labor. Thus, the provision of social support to reduce maternal anxiety should promote raised levels of uterine contractibility, shorter duration labor, and a reduced rate of complications requiring Caesarian or forceps delivery; such complications are more common when labor is prolonged and uterine contractibility is reduced. A positive chain of events of this sort has been postulated by researchers such as Klaus and seems physiologically probable. However, it remains to be conclusively demonstrated.

Overall, then, it would appear that the effects of social support may be realized through a number of mechanisms. Healthy behaviors may be increased, material benefits may accrue and the physiological impact of psychological stress may be attenuated. However, it must be noted that many of these studies are correlational in nature and so the precise causal path is difficult to establish. Thus, for instance those who indulge in healthy behaviors may attract more social support, rather than support promoting the behaviors.

SOCIAL SUPPORT AND GENDER

The second question we posed is why social support appears to exert less of an effect for women. Why, particularly in the mortality studies, are the effects more pronounced for men?

One possible explanation lies in the power of many of these studies to detect effects. Although the sample sizes in all the prospective studies reviewed earlier were large, some may still have had insufficient power to detect effects for women, given their low levels of mortality relative to men. This is a point made cogently in an earlier chapter by Light and Girdler. In the current context, it is perhaps worth noting that the two studies with the largest sample sizes (Berkman and Syme, 1979; Orth-Gomer and Johnson, 1987) do report social support effects for the bulk of women that are similar to those recorded for men. However, in the Orth-Gomer and Johnson (1987) study, larger social networks in older women were associated with higher rates of mortality.

There may also be genuine differences in the dynamics of social networks for men and women that have implications for the relative health benefits that accrue. As Shumaker and Hill (1991) pointed out, women tend to have less extensive but more intensive networks than men. Women, for example, are more likely than men to have confidants. The absence of a confidant would seem to be especially characteristic of men in low status occupations (Marmot *et al.*, 1991). In addition, women's networks appear to be more multifaceted than men's.

However, it is in the provision of social support rather than in its reception that the most marked gender differences appear. Kessler *et al.* (1985) reported that women were 30 percent more likely than men to provide support to network members. Not only do men rely more on women as their primary source of social support but so too, in the main, do women. In general, women are more likely to be involved in all forms of helping and care-giving. It is not just that they are more frequent providers of informal support; they also dominate in formal care-giving settings such as nursing and social work. Thus, as Shumaker and Hill (1991) pithily stated, women often give at the office as well as at home.

Unfortunately, there has been considerably more research on the consequences of receiving support than on the effects of giving it. Nevertheless, there is now at least preliminary evidence that excessive support demands can have deleterious effects on mental and physical well-being. For example, Light and Lebowitz (1988) reported relatively high rates of depression among Alzheimer's disease care-givers. Further comparisons between such care-givers and matched control subjects revealed the former to be much more distressed and have significantly poorer immune function than the latter (Kiecolt-Glaser *et al.*, 1987a).

Thus, it might be conjectured that as women's social networks expand so the demands upon them as expected providers of care and support increase (see Belle, 1982). Accordingly, while men would be expected to benefit from an expansion of their social networks because the balance of interaction for them would favor the receiving over the giving of support, for women the reverse would hold. For women, increases in social contact will most likely mean extra demands for support, such that any of the health benefits that seem to follow directly for men would be offset by the strains incumbent on increased helping and giving.

MARRIAGE, GENDER AND HEALTH

There is evidence that the extent of social networks is relatively less important than the quality of support provided. The majority of studies which examine the relationship between quality and quantity of social support and positive outcomes indicate that quality of support is the more critical variable (see, eg. Antonucci, 1985). Marriage can clearly be one of the most intimate of social relationships and evidence indicates that marriage affords substantial advantage in terms of both mortality and morbidity. Those who are not married, whether single, divorced or widowed, register higher mortality rates than those who are (see, eg. Berkman, 1985). Morbidity in a variety of areas is similarly reduced by marriage (see, eg. Blaxter, 1987). However, in both cases the advantage conferred by marriage is substantially greater for men than it is for women.

Helsing *et al.* (1981) examined mortality rates among 4032 male and female adult residents of Washington Country, Maryland who were widowed between 1963 and 1974. These cases and matched married control subjects were followed up until 1975. Being widowed was found to increase significantly the mortality risk for men but not for women. In addition, this increased risk for men persisted when age, education, cigarette smoking and economic status, among other variables, were controlled for. Finally, increased risk was spread across a range of mortality courses. In the UK, Fox and Goldblatt (1982), calculated standardized mortality ratios from one percent of the 1971 population census. Married men and women registered substantially lower values than single, divorced or widowed men and women. However, the difference between being single and being married was less for women than it was for men at all ages.

While there are less large scale data available on marital status and self-reported and physician-assessed physical morbidity what there are seem to point in the same general direction. For example, the British Health and Life-style Survey (Blaxter, 1987) contrasted illness scores of people over 60, either living alone or with their spouses. For women, difference in status had only a marginal influence on illness, whereas for men those living with a spouse enjoyed substantially better scores than those living alone. Macintyre (1986) reported a study in which married men in all age groups between 30 and 70 registered better health in the previous year than single men, whereas no such consistent pattern emerged for women. Mental health also appears to be affected by marital status in much the same way (see, eg. Cochrane, 1983). While the married have lower rates of mental hospital admission than the single, divorced or widowed, the difference in rates between the married and the unmarried is much less for women than it is for men.

If marriage represents a major source of social support for most people, the greater relative health advantage it affords men may derive, at least in part, from the usual distribution of social support within marriage, ie. that more support in marriage flows from women to men than vice-versa. There is evidence in accord with this contention. For example, Belle (1982) reported a study of help seeking among working class husbands and wives which revealed that husbands were more inclined to seek support from their wives than vice-versa. Campbell *et al.* (1976) observed that husbands were more likely than wives to report that their spouses understood them well, and wives more likely than husbands to report that they understood their spouses well. The following *cri de couer* recorded by Miles (1988) undoubtedly typifies the lot of many married women "My husband is there but he doesn't want to talk. He doesn't understand. He just says 'don't bother me'." (p.95).

It is also possible that, in addition to gaining less satisfactory social support within marriage, women are more adversely affected by marital dissatisfaction than men. Two recent studies suggest that this notion is worthy of further exploration. Kiecolt-Glaser *et al.* (1987b) monitored immunological function in 38 married women and 38 comparable separated or divorced women. All of this latter group had been separated within the last six years and 16 of them had been separated within the last year. In addition, the married group were administered a questionnaire to assess their perceptions of the quality of their marriage. Those women who had been separated for one year or less were revealed to have poorer immune functioning. Importantly in the present context, for the married women, it was observed that the poorer the self-reported quality of marriage, the greater the level of psychological distress and the less the immune reaction to an introduced antigen. In a study of hypertensive men and women, Ewart *et al.* (1991) measured blood pressure reactions to two sorts of communications with their partners, neutral conversation and disagreement. As might be expected, blood pressures overall were more elevated in the latter condition. However, women displayed a greater elevation in systolic blood pressure during disagreements than men, and for women, but not men, larger magnitude systolic blood pressure reactions were associated with greater marital dissatisfaction. Taken together, these studies suggest that marital discord may be particularly pathogenic for women. During pregnancy and after birth, a poor marital relationship may have a particularly marked effect on levels of depression in women. Scott-Heyes (1984) found that women who received little affection and nurturance from their husband during pregnancy were more likely to be depressed at that time. This pattern continued after the birth and has also been found in studies of post-natal depression (Elliot *et al.*, 1988; Holden *et al.*, 1989) and post-natal emotional distress (Ball, 1989).

For many men marriage represents a consolidation and even intensification of their existing social relations, whereas for many women it represents a curtailment. Gove and Tudor (1973), for example, pointed out that most married men usually have two major social roles from which they may draw satisfaction and support: their role within the household and their role at work. In contrast, married women without paid employment outside the home have to rely on but one potential source of support. Accordingly, the differential health advantages conferred on men by marriage may have something to do with their continuation in employment, a facility that is denied many married women, particularly following the birth of children.

It is, perhaps, worth noting that in this context women at home with children are particularly vulnerable to a range of physical and mental health problems (Arber *et al.*, 1985; Brown and Harris, 1978). While children certainly provide 'comfort, caring and esteem' for their parents, the nature of the parent/child relation is more generally characterized by the parental provision of emotional and material support. Although men are generally more involved in parenting than they were in the past, recent research clearly demonstrates that baby and child care is still predominantly 'women's work' (see Niven, 1992, for a review). Earlier we argued that support in marriage more often flows from women to men. Similarly, the flow of social support is more likely to be from mother to child than vice versa. Accordingly, wives and mothers may be considered to be doubly disadvantaged. In addition, children at times may act as a source of social undermining or destruction; think for example of the crying, sleep-depriving baby, or the hostile adolescent. Finally, mothers in paid employment most likely work 'double shifts', ie. they work at work and work at home. Evidence of the potentially destructive effects of such overload comes from a recent study of white collar Volvo workers in Sweden (Frankenhaeuser *et al.*, 1989). Male and female participants performed the same job between 9 and 5 p.m.. However, whereas men were assessed as completing a total average workload (combining paid and unpaid domestic work) of 68 hours per week, women tallied 78 hours and this figure increased with increases in the number of children living at home. Gender differences in physiological arousal during the working day were small. However, in the evening male noradrenaline (norepinephrine) levels dropped sharply, whereas female levels continued to rise. Frankenhaeuser (1991) concluded from these data that whereas male managers wound down in the evening, female managers wound up.

WOMEN, PAID EMPLOYMENT AND HEALTH

The foregoing discussion raises the issue of whether paid employment outside the home *per se* may advantage or disadvantage health. There is now substantial evidence, particularly from studies examining the effects of involuntary unemployment (see, eg. Warr, 1987), that employment is broadly health promoting. In addition, recent research focussing specifically on women indicates that paid employment outside the home brings benefits both for mortality and morbidity.

Passannante and Nathanson (1985) examined the death certificates of women in Wisconsin and found that for younger and middle-aged women (ie. under 60 years of age), the mortality rate for housewives was approximately twice as high as that of employed women. In terms of morbidity, the evidence points with unerring consistency in the same direction (see LaCroix and Haynes, 1987). For example, Haavio-Mannila (1986), in a study conducted using data from four Scandinavian countries, examined the overall pattern of morbidity and specific symptoms of anxiety in wives and husbands, both in households where wives worked in paid employment and in households where they did not. Anxiety was included as an outcome measure because it was considered to be a good index of stress. A consistent pattern of effects characterized all four countries. Gender inequalities in morbidity and anxiety symptomatology were much greater when women stayed at home; paid employment outside the home made women much healthier. In addition, women's employment status had no negative impact on their husband's morbidity or anxiety. Finally, paid employment among women would not seem to be associated with increases in unhealthy behavior; neither smoking patterns (Waldron and Lye, 1989) nor alcohol problems (Wilsnack and Cheloha, 1987) are affected.

For some, such results appear counter-intuitive (see, eg. Miles, 1991). Since it remains the case that women in paid employment shoulder the bulk of domestic responsibilities, it might be suspected that such multiplicity of demands could lead to what has been labeled 'role overload' (see Cochrane, in Chapter 9 for a discussion of this concept). Given our previous contention that an expansion of support networks might overextend women, because of their primacy as providers of support and care, the suspicion arises that additional social demands contingent on employment could contribute to stress. We have also seen that women derive far less benefit from marriage than men and, in part, this may stem from the particular strains attendant on working women with children at home. In fact, Miles (1991) has argued that the mortality and morbidity data reported earlier could arise from an artefact, in that women suffering from chronic sickness or disability that impedes their employability prefer to describe themselves as just housewives. Thus, health comparisons of women with or without paid employment outside the home would be biased by the inclusion of those unavailable for work as a result of sickness or disability in the latter category. However, the available evidence does not favor this sort of explanation. In the San Antonio Heart Study, employment status was examined in terms of cardiovascular disease risk factors. The health advantage of employed women persisted, even when all women with any history of chronic disease or disability were excluded (Hazuda *et al.*, 1986). As Cochrane eloquently points out, the concept of role overload has not faired well and the evidence cited above is but illustrative of a general absence of empirical support.

What functions might work be serving that renders it beneficial to women's health. The most obvious benefit is the financial one. As Belle (1982) observed, "If money cannot buy love, it can buy health sustaining relief from otherwise overwhelming demands." (p.501). We have already alluded to the impact of economic support. Its importance in the context of work is apparent from a study by Arber *et al.* (1985), where the benefits of employment for self-reported health were observed to vary with occupational status. Women whose jobs were managerial or professional reported much less ill-health than women in manual or low-level non-manual jobs; only the former were advantaged over women remaining at home. Rodin and Ickovics (1990) reported similar findings. Women who felt that they were poorly paid and under-utilized in their jobs registered worse physical and mental health than women with adequate employment. Undoubtedly, women in better paid employment have the material resources to alleviate the burdens of housework and childcare, thus reducing the stresses that such responsibilities can bring.

Nevertheless, it is unlikely that material factors afford a complete explanation. Arnetz *et al.* (1987) examined immune function in a sample of recently unemployed Swedish women and a comparable control group of women in stable employment. Since those unemployed were in receipt of full benefit, ie. 90 percent of their previous income under the Swedish welfare system, financial penalty was not an issue. Blood samples were taken at various intervals during the first 12 months of unemployment and at comparable times for the control subjects. After nine months of unemployment, immune reaction to an antigen was observed to decrease for the unemployed women, whereas the employed no such reduction was apparent.

Work fulfils other complex social functions. Jahoda and Rush (1980) listed five such functions, which they argued were only properly satisfied by paid employment, ie. charitable work or leisure activities might fulfil some of these functions but could not satisfy all of them. First of all, work imposes a definitive time structure on the day. Second, work demands social contact and third, it requires that the individual cooperates with these contacts in order to achieve collective goals. Fourth, work confers an identity and social status on an individual. Fifthly, work requires people to be active. Additionally, work may act as a potent distractor as research on coping with chronic pain has demonstrated (Wynn Parry, 1980).

These social aspects of work may be crucial in either offsetting inherent job stress or in compensating for stress and impoverished social relations in other aspects of life. For example, Miles (1991) reported that the positive association between employment and health was most marked among women with the least access to opportunities for deriving support and esteem in the domestic context. Johnson (1986) examined the effects of various occupational parameters on cardiovascular disease prevalence. While high demand at work was associated with increased disease prevalence for both men and women, its effects were very much mitigated by a combination of good relations with co-workers and the capacity to exercise control at work. This facility for control may to an extent underlie Arber *et al.*'s (1985) results (see above).

CONCLUDING REMARKS

In this chapter we have examined a number of broad social factors that might contribute to the different patterns of mortality and morbidity experienced by women and men. It has to be conceded, though, that the available evidence in this context yields, at best, only partial answers to the apparent paradox of women's greater morbidity but reduced mortality. While psychosocial stress and the nature of social relations may be important factors in the health inequalities attendant on material division (Wilkinson, 1992), their contributions to gender variation are more difficult to discern.

It would seem to be the case that both men and women benefit from better material provision (Whitehead, 1988) and that both benefit from paid employment, particularly where it is financially, personally and socially rewarding. If anything, however, men appear to derive greater advantage from expanded social networks than women and almost certainly derive greater benefits from marriage. It is possible that this shortfall in social relations' dividends contributes something to women's higher morbidity rates as does their greater experience of psychosocial stress. However, we are still left with the puzzle of women's substantially lower rates of mortality. Further, for specific diseases, one gender usually has both higher morbidity and mortality rates (Verbrugge and Wingard, 1987). For example, men not only have higher death rates for cardiovascular disease, they also have higher rates of morbidity; coronary heart disease alone accounts for over 40 percent of the gender difference in mortality in the US and UK.

One is left with the almost inescapable conclusion that as far as 'killer' afflictions, such as cardiovascular disease, are concerned, women are simply less prone than men. As indicated in Chapter 1, gender differences in unhealthy behaviors account for only a portion of the variation in cardiovascular disease mortality. It has been argued that as the relative incidence of cigarette smoking and alcohol consumption increases among women, so gender mortality rates will converge (Rodin and Ickovics, 1990). However, while there is a temporal lag in the realizability of such effects, the epidemiological evidence favors caution. In most Western countries, unhealthy behavior has increased in women while it has declined in men. However, in general, the striking gender differentials in cardiovascular disease mortality and overall mortality rates remain. Where a temporal change in overall life expectancy relativities can be detected, it is generally in the form of a 'leveling off': a consolidation of women's life expectancy advantage over men at around six or seven years. Even in Japan, where people now have the longest life expectancy in the world, women still enjoy this order of advantage. Only in 'non-developed' countries can exceptions to this pattern be discerned and this almost certainly reflects risks attendant on childbearing (see, eg. Verbrugge and Wingard, 1987).

Rodin and Ickovics (1990) concluded their review of women's health by plotting a broad agendum for research. It included the following: increased inclusion of women in the study populations of health research; increased attention to the health concerns that uniquely or predominantly affect women; greater emphasis on gender comparative research; more attention to women's health as a function of their ethnicity and social and material circumstances; greater concern with women's health across the life cycle. We are more than happy to endorse such an agendum. Nevertheless, it is important not to lose sight of women's essential hardiness. In spite of high levels of morbidity, women persist in substantially outliving men. So perhaps we should conclude by celebrating women's resilience. However, for many women such relative longevity remains a mixed blessing; many have to deal with bereavement, with having to spend a substantial period towards the end of their lives without close companionship in reduced material circumstances, and with having to cope with declining health and increasing incapacity.

FURTHER READING

Cohen, S. and Syme, S.L. (1985). *Social support and health*. New York: Academic Press.
Shumaker, S.A. and Hill, D.R. (1991). Gender differences in social support and physical health. *Health Psychology*, 10, 102–111.
Whitehead, M. (1988). *The health divide*. Harmondsworth: Penguin.

REFERENCES

Adams, M.R., Kaplan, J.R., Clarkson, T.B. and Koritnik, D.R. (1985). Ovariectomy, social status, and atherosclerosis in cynomolgus monkeys. *Arteriosclerosis*, 5, 192–200.

Adib, T. (1988). Opinions about medical procedures: media and framing effects. Unpublished BSc thesis, University of London.

Adler, N.E., David, H.P., Major, B.N., Roth, S.H., Russo, N.F. and Wyatt, G.E. (1990). Psychological responses after abortion. *Science*, 248, 41–44.

Adler, N.E., Keyes, S. and Robertson, P. (1991). Psychological issues in new reproductive technologies: pregnancy–inducing technology and diagnostic screening. In J. Rodin and A. Collins (Eds.), *Women and new reproductive technology: Medical, psychosocial, legal and ethical dilemmas.* Hillsdale, NJ: Lawrence Erlbaum.

Alder, E., Cook, A., Gray, J., Tyrer, G., Warner, P. and Bancroft, J. (1981). The effects of sterilisation: a comparison of sterilised women with the wives of vasectomised men. *Contraception*, 23, 45–54.

Alder, E. (1984a). Psychological aspects of AID. In I. Pullen and A.H. Emery (Eds.), *Pschological aspects of genetic counselling.* London: Academic Press.

Alder, E. (1984b). Sterilization. In A. Broome and L. Wallace (Eds.), *Psychology and gynaecological problems* London: Tavistock.

Alder, E. (1989). Sexual behaviour in pregnancy, after childbirth and during breast feeding. In M.R. Oates (Ed.), *Psychological aspects of obstetrics and gynaecology Bailliere's clinical obstetrics and gynaecology 3 no 4.* London: Bailliere Tindall.

Allen, K.M., Blascovich, J., Tomaka, J., and Kelsey, R.M. (1991). Presence of human friends and pet dogs as moderators of autonomic responses to stress in women. *Journal of Personality and Social Psychology*, 61, 582–589.

Alter-Reid, K., Gibbs, M.S., Lachenmeyer, J.R., Signal, J., and Massoth, N.A. (1986). Sexual abuse of children: a review of the empirical findings. *Clinical Psychology Review*, 6, 249–266.

American Cancer Society (1992). *Cancer facts and figures – 1992.* New York: American Cancer Society.

Amery, A., Brixko, R., Clement, D., de Schaepdryver, A., Fagard, R., Torte, J., Henry, J.F., Leonetti, G., O'Malley, K., Straser, T., Birkenhager, W., Bulpitt, C., Deruyttere, M., Dollery, C., Forette, F., Hamdy, R., Joossens, J.V., Lund–Johansen, P., Petrie, J. and Tuomilehto, J. (1985). Mortality and morbidity results from the European working party on high blood pressure in the elderly trial. *Lancet*, 1, 1349–1354.

Anastos, K., Charney, P., Charon, R.A., Cohen, E., Jones, C.Y., Marte, C., Swiderski, D.M., Wheat, M.E. and Williams, S. (1991). Hypertension in women: What is really known? Report of The Women's Caucus, Working Group on Women's Health of the Society of General Internal Medicine. *Annals of Internal Medicine*, 115, 287–293.

Andersch, B., Wendestam, C., Hahn, L. and Ohman, R. (1986). Premenstrual complaints. I. Prevalence of premenstrual symptoms in a Swedish urban population. *Journal of Psychosomatic Obstetrics and Gynaecology*, 5, 39–49.

Andersen, B.L. (1985). Sexual functioning morbidity among cancer survivors. Present status and future research directions. *Cancer*, 55, 1835–1842.

Andersen, B.L. (in press). Predicting sexual and psychological morbidity and improving quality of life for women with gynecologic cancer. *Cancer.*

171

Andersen, B.L. (in press). Psychological interventions for cancer patients. *Journal of Consulting and Clinical Psychology*.

Andersen, B.L., Anderson, B. and deProsse, C. (1989a). Controlled prospective longitudinal study of women with cancer: I. Sexual functioning outcomes. *Journal of Consulting and Clinical Psychology*, **57**, 683–691.

Andersen, B.L., Anderson, B. and deProsse, C. (1989b). Controlled prospective longitudinal study of women with cancer: II. Psychological outcomes. *Journal of Consulting and Clinical Psychology*, **57**, 692–697.

Andersen, B.L. and Hacker, N.F. (1983). Psychosexual adjustment after vulvar surgery. *Obstetrics and Gynecology*, **62**, 457–462.

Andersen, B.L., Karlsson, J.A., Anderson, B. and Tewfik, H.H. (1984). Anxiety and cancer treatment: Response to stressful radiotherapy. *Health Psychology*, **3**, 535–551.

Andersen, B.L. and Tewfik, H.H. (1985). Psychological reactions to radiation therapy: Reconsideration of the adaptive aspects of anxiety. *Journal of Personality and Social Psychology*, **48**, 1024–1032.

Anderson, L., Aspegren, K., Janzon, L., Landberg, T., Lindholm, K., Linell, F., Ljungberg, O., Ranstan, T. and Sigfusson, B. (1988). Mammographic screening and mortality from breast cancer: the Malmo mammographic screening trial. *British Medical Journal*, **297**, 943–948.

Anderson, W. (1991). The New York Needle Trial: The politics of public health in the age of AIDS. *American Journal of Public Health*, **81**, 1506–1517.

Andiman, W.A. and Modlin, J.F. (1991). Vertical transmission. In P.A. Pizzo and C.M. Wilfert (Eds.), *Pediatric AIDS*. Baltimore, MD: Williams and Wilkins.

Antonucci, T.C. (1985). Social support: Theoretical advances, recent findings and pressing issues. In I.G. Sarason and B. Sarason (Eds.). *Social Support: Theory, research and applications.* The Hague, Netherlands: Martinus Nijhoff.

Arber, S. (1989). Gender and class inequalities in health: Understanding the differentials. In J. Fox (Ed.) *Health inequalities in European countries.* Aldershot: Gower Publishing Co.

Arber, S., Gilbert, G.N. and Dale, A. (1985). Paid employment and women's health: A benefit or a source of role strain? *Sociology of Health and Illness*, **7**, 375–400.

Arnetz, B.B., Wasserman, J., Petrini, B., Brenner, S–O., Levi, L., Eneroth, P., Salovaara, H., Hjelm, R., Salovaara, L., Theorell, T. and Petterson, I–L. (1987). Immune function in unemployed women. *Psychosomatic Medicine*, **49**, 3–11.

Asso, D. (1983). *The real menstrual cycle*. Chichester: Wiley.

Astbury, J. (1980) Labour pain: the role of childbirth education, information and education. In C. Peck and M Wallace (Eds.). *Problems in pain*. London: Pergamon.

Austoker, J., Humphries, J., and Roberts, M.M. (1989). *Breast cancer screening, Scottish edition, practical guides for general practice*. Oxford: Oxford University Press.

Baider, L. and Sarell, M. (1984). Couples in crisis: Patient-spouse differences in perception of interaction patterns and the illness situation. *Family Therapy*, **11**, 115–122.

Ball, J. (1989). Postnatal care and adjustment to motherhood. In S. Robinson and A.M. Thomson (Eds.), *Midwives, research and childbirth. Volume 1*. London: Chapman and Hall.

Bancroft, J. and Backstrom, T. (1985). Premenstrual syndrome. *Clinical Endocrinology*, **22**, 313–336.

Bancroft, J., Cook, A., Davidson, D., Bennie, J. and Goodwin, G. (1991). Blunting of neuroendocrine response to infusion of L-tryptophan in women with perimenstrual mood change. *Psychological Medicine*, **21**, 305–312.

Bancroft, J., Williamson, L., Warner, P., Rennie, D. and Smith, S. (1992). Perimenstrual complaints in women complaining of PMS, menorrhagia and dysmenorrhoea: Towards a dismantling of the 'premenstrual syndrome' (submitted for publication).

Bandura, A. (1977). Self-efficacy: Towards a unifying theory of behavioral change. *Psychological Review*, **84**, 191–215.

Bard, M. and Sutherland, A.M. (1952). Adaptation to radical mastectomy. *Cancer*, **8**, 656–671.

Barefoot, J.C., Peterson, B.L., Dahlstrom, W.G., Siegler, I.C., Anderson, N.B. and Williams, R.B. (1991). Hostility patterns and health implications: Correlates of Cooke-Medley hostility scale scores in a national survey. *Health Psychology*, 10, 18–24.

Barnett, R.C. and Baruch, G.K. (1985). Women's involvement in multiple roles and psychological distress. *Journal of Personality and Social Psychology*, 49, 135–145.

Baum, A. and Grunberg, N.E. (1991). Gender, stress and health. *Health Psychology*, 10, 80–85.

Baum, C., Kennedy, D.L., Knapp, D.E., Juergens, J.P. and Faich, G.A. (1988). Prescription drug use in 1984 and changes over time. *Medical Care*, 26, 105–114.

Bean, J. (1986). Epidemiologic review of cancer in women. In B.L. Andersen (Ed.), *Women with cancer: Psychological perspectives*, New York: Springer-Verlag.

Bean, J.D., Clark, M.P. and South, S. (1982). Changes in sexual desire after voluntary sterilization. *Social Biology* 27, 186–193.

Beck, A.T. (1976). *Cognitive therapy and the emotional disorders*. New York: International Universities Press.

Becker, J.V., Skinner, L.J. and Abel, G.G. (1983). Sequelae of sexual assault: The survivor's perspective. In J.G. Greer and I.R. Stuart (Eds.) *The sexual aggressor*. New York: Van Nostrand.

Becker, M.H., Haefner, D.P., Kals, S.V., Kirscht, J.P., Maiman, L.A. and Rosenstock, I.M. (1977). Selected psychosocial models and correlates of individual health-related behaviours. *Medical Care*, 15, 27–46.

Becker, M.H., Maiman, L.A., Kirscht, J.P., Haefner, D.P. and Drachman, R.H. (1977). The health belief model and prediction of dietary compliance: A field experiment. *Journal of Health and Social Behavior*, 18, 348–366.

Belle, D. (1982). The stress of caring: Women as providers of social support. In L. Goldberger and S. Bruntz (Eds.). *Handbook of stress: Theoretical and clinical aspects*. New York: Free Press.

Bennett, P. and Carroll, D. (1990). Type A behaviours and heart disease: Epidemiological and experimental foundations. *Behavioural Neurology*, 3, 261–277.

Bentler, P.M. and Newcomb, M.D. (1978). Longitudinal study of marital success and failure. *Journal of Consulting and Clinical Psychology*, 46, 1053–1070.

Beral, V., Peterman, T.A., Berkelman, R.L. and Jaffe, H.W. (1990). Kaposki's sarcoma among persons with AIDS: a sexually transmitted infection? *The Lancet*, 335, 123–128.

Berkman, L.F. (1991). Social support and cardiovascular disease morbidity and mortality in women. Paper presented at the National Heart, Lung and Blood Institute Conference on Women, Behavior and Cardiovascular Disease, Chevy Chase, MD, September 25–27, 1991.

Berlinger E., Melzack, R. and Lauzon, P. (1989) Pain of first-trimester abortion: a study of psychosocial and medical predictors. *Pain*, 36, 339–350.

Berryman, J. (1991). Perspectives on later motherhood. In A. Phoenix, A. Woollett and E. Lloyd (Eds.), *Motherhood, meanings, practices and ideologies*, London: Sage.

Bielawska-Batorowicz, E. (1990). Attitudes to motherhood of women in high-risk and normal pregnancy. *Journal of Reproductive and Infant Psychology*, 8, 3–9.

Blair, A.J., Booth, D.A., Lewis, V.J. and Wainwright, C.J. (1989). The relative success of official and informal weight reduction techniques: Retrospective correlational evidence. *Psychology and Health*, 3, 195–206.

Blanchard, C.G., Ruckdeschel, J.C., Labrecque, M.S., Frisch, S. and Blanchard, E.B. (1987). The impact of a designated cancer unit on house staff behaviors toward patients. Cancer, 60, 2348–2354.

Blandford, G.F. (1871). *Insanity and its treatment*. Philadelphia: Henry C. Lea.

Blaxter, M. (1987). Self-reported health. In B.D. Cox (Ed.), *The health and life-style survey*. London: Health-Promotion Research Trust.

Blaxter, M. (1989). A comparison of measures of inequality in morbidity. In J. Fox (Ed.), *Health inequalities in European countries.* Aldershot: Gower Publishing Co.

Blaxter, M. (1990). Health and lifestyle. Tavistock: London.

Bloom, J.R. (1987). Psychological response to mastectomy. *Cancer*, 59, 189–196.

Blumenthal, J.A., Burg, M.M., Barefoot, J., Williams, R.B., Honey, T. and Zimet, C. (1987). Social support, Type A behavior, and coronary artery disease. *Psychosomatic Medicine*, 49, 331–339.

Bonica, J.J. (1984). Pain research and therapy: recent advances and future needs. In: L. Kruger and J. Liebeskind (Eds.). *Advances in pain research and therapy (vol. 6) Neural mechanisms of pain.* Raven Press: New York.

Bonime, W. (1976). The psychodynamics of neurotic depression. *Journal of American Academy of Psychoanalysis.* 4, 301–326.

Bontekoe, E.H.M., Blacquiere, J.F., Naaktgeboren, C., Dieleman, S.J. and Willems, P.P.M. (1977). Influence of environmental disturbances on uterine motility during pregnancy and parturition in rabbit and sheep. *Behavioural Processes*, 2, 41–73.

Boorse, C. (1987). Premenstrual syndrome and criminal responsibility. In B.E. Ginsburg and B.F. Carter (Eds.), *Ethical and legal implications in a biomedical perspective.* New York: Plenum.

Booth, R., Koester, S., Brewster, J.T., Weibel, W.W. and Fritz, R.B. (1991). Intravenous drug users and AIDS: Risk behaviors. *American Journal of Drug and Alcohol Abuse*, 17, 337–353.

Borghi, C., Costa, F.V., Boschi, S., Mussi, A. and Ambrosioni, E. (1986). Predictors of stable hypertension in young borderline subjects: A five-year follow-up study. *Journal of Cardiovascular Pharmacology*, 8 (Suppl. 5), S138–S141.

Boring, C.C., Squires, T.S. and Tong, T. (1992). Cancer statistics, 1992. *Ca – A Cancer Journal for Clinicians*, 42, 19–38.

Bromham, D.R., Bryce, F.C., Balmer, B. and Wright, S. (1989). Psychometric evaluation of infertile couples: (preliminary findings). *Journal of Reproductive and Infant Psychology*, 7, 195–202.

Brook, S.J. and Smith, C. (1991). Do combined oral contraceptive users know how to take their contraceptive pill correctly? *British Journal of Family Planning*, 17, 18–20.

Brown, R. (1991, January). AIDS: The growing threat to black heterosexuals. *Ebony*, pp. 84, 86, 88, 90.

Brown, G.R. and Rundell, J.R. (1990). Prospective study of psychiatric morbidity in HIV-seropositive women without AIDS. *General Hospital Psychiatry*, 12, 30–35.

Brown, G.R. and Rundell, J.R. (in press). Prospective study of psychiatric aspects of early HIV infection in women. *American Journal of Psychiatry.*

Brown, G.W. and Harris, T.O. (1973). *Social origins of depression: a study of psychiatric disorder in women.* London: Tavistock.

Bruch, M.A. and Haynes, M.J. (1987). Heterosexual anxiety and contraceptive behaviour. *Journal of Research in Personality*, 21: 343–60.

Bryer, J.B., Nelson, B.A., Miller, J.B. and Krol, P.A. (1987). Childhood sexual and physical abuse as factors in adult psychiatric illness. *American Journal of Psychiatry*, 144, 1426–1430.

Burish, T.G. and Redd, W.H. (1983). Behavioral approaches to reducing conditioned responses to chemotherapy in adult cancer patients. *Behavioral Medicine Update*, 5, 12–16.

Cain, E.N., Kohorn, E.I., Quinlan, D.M., Latimer, K. and Schwartz, P.E. (1986). Psychosocial benefits of a cancer support group. *Cancer*, 57, 183–189.

Calnan, M., (1984). The Health Belief Model and participation in programmes for the early detection of breast cancer: A comparative analysis. *Social Science and Medicine*, 19, 823–830.

Campbell, A., Converse, P. and Rodgers, W. (1976). *The quality of American life: Perceptions, evaluations, and satisfactions.* New York: Russell Sage.

Campbell, C.A. (1990). Prostitution and AIDS. In D.G. Ostrow (Ed.), *Behavioral aspects of AIDS.* New York: Plenum.

Campbell, E. (1985). *The Childless Marriage.* London: Tavistock.

Canino, G.J., Rubro–Stipec, M., Shrout, P., Bravo, M., Stolberg, R. and Bird, H.R. (1987). Sex differences and depression in Puerto Rico. *Psychology of Women Quarterly*, 11, 443–459.

Cannon, W.B. (1935). Stresses and strains of homeostasis. *American Journal of Medical Sciences*, 189, 1–14.

Capone, M.A., Good, R.S., Westie, K.S. and Jacobson, A.F. (1980). Psychosocial rehabilitation of gynecologic oncology patients. *Archives of Physical Medicine and Rehabilitation*, 61, 128–132.

Carey, M.P. and Burish, T.G. (1988). Etiology and treatment of the psychological side effects associated with cancer chemotherapy. *Psychological Bulletin*, 104, 307–325.

Carmen, E., Russon, N.F. and Miller, J.B. (1981). Inequality and women's mental health: an overview. *American Journal of Psychiatry*, 138, 1319–1330.

Carney, R.M. (1991). Depression and negative affect as cardiovascular disease risk factors in women. Paper presented at the National Heart, Lung and Blood Institute Conference on Women, Behavior and Cardiovascular Disease, Chevy Chase, MD, September 25–27, 1991.

Carney, R.M., Rich, M.W. and Freedland, K.E. (1989). Psychiatric depression, anxiety and coronary heart disease. *Comprehensive Therapy*, 15, 8–13.

Carpenter, C.C.J., Mayer, K.H., Stein, M.D., Leibman, B.D., Fisher, A. and Fiore, T.C. (1991). Human immunodefiency virus infection in North American women: Experience with 200 cases and a review of the literature. *Medicine*, 70, 307–325.

Carroll, D., Harris, M.G. and Cross, G. (1991). Haemodynamic adjustments to mental stress in normotensives and subjects with mildly elevated blood pressure. *Psychophysiology*, 28, 439–447.

Carroll, D., Hewitt, J.K., Last, K., Turner, J.R. and Sims, J. (1985). A twin study of cardiac reactivity and its relationship to parental blood pressure. *Physiology and Behavior*, 34, 103–106.

Cartwright, A. (1987). Trends in family intentions and the use of contraception among recent mothers, 1967–84. *Population Trends*, 49, 31–34.

Cassileth, B.R., Lusk, E.J., Strouse, T.B., Miller, D.S., Brown, L.L. and Cross, P.A. (1985). A psychological analysis of cancer patients and their next-of-kin. *Cancer*, 55, 72–76.

Cassileth, P.A. and Cassileth, B.R. (1983a, March). Clinical care of the terminal cancer patient: Part I. *Medical Times*, March, 57s–66s.

Cassileth, P.A. and Cassileth, B.R. (1983b, April). Clinical care of the terminal cancer patient: Part II. *Medical Times*, March, 9s–22s.

CDC AIDS Weekly. (1991, August). p. 2.

Cella, D.F. and Tross, S. (1986). Psychological adjustment to survival from Hodgkin's Disease. *Journal of Consulting and Clinical Psychology*, 54, 616–622.

Centers for Disease Control. (1985). Recommendations for assisting in the prevention of perinatal transmission of human T. lymphotrophic virus type III/lymphadenopathy associated virus and acquired immunodeficiency syndrome. *Morbidity and Mortality Weekly Report*, 36, 721–726, 731–732.

Centers for Disease Control. (1987, August). Revision of the CDC surveillance case definition for acquired immunodeficiency syndrome. *Morbidity and Mortality Weekly Report*, 36(1S), 3S–15S.

Centers for Disease Control. (1989, May). *HIV/AIDS Surveillance Report*, pp. 1–14. Atlanta GA: Centers for Disease Control.

Centers for Disease Control. (1989). Guidelines for prophylaxis against *Pneumocystis carinii* pneumonia for persons infected with human immunodeficiency virus. *Morbidity and Mortality Weekly Report*, 38(S-5), 1–9.

Centers for Disease Control (1990, October). HIV/AIDS *Surveillance Report*, 1–18 Atlanta, GA: Centers for Disease Control.

Centers for Disease Control. (1990, December). Current trends: AIDS in women – United States. *Morbidity and Mortality Weekly Report*, 39, 845–846.

Centers for Disease Control. (1990). *National HIV Seroprevalence surveys* – summary of results: Data from serosurveillance activities through 1989. Atlanta: US Department of Health and Human Services, Public Health Service, DHHS Publication no. (CDC)HIV/CID/9-90/006.

Centers for Disease Control. (1991, October). *HIV/AIDS Surveillance Report*, 1-18. Atlanta, GA: Centers for Disease Control.

Chan, Y.F., O'Hoy, K.M., Wong So, W.K., Ho, P.C. and Tsoi M.M. (1989). Psychosocial evaluation in an IVF/GIFT program in Hong Kong. *Journal of Reproductive and Infant Psychology*, 7, 67-77.

Chaudhary, N.A. and Truelove, S.C. (1962). The irritable colon syndrome: A study of the clinical features, predisposing causes and prognosis in 130 cases. *Quarterly Journal of Medicine*, 3, 307-332.

Chavkin W., Cohen J., Ehrhardt A., Fullilove M. and Worth, D. (1991). Women and AIDS. *Science*, 251, 359-360.

Chin, J. (1990). Current and future dimensions of the HIV/AIDS pandemic in women and children. *Lancet*, 336, 221-224.

Chin, J. (1990, November–December). Challenge of the nineties. *World Health*, pp. 4-6.

Chirgwin, K., DeHovitz, J.A., Dillon, S. and McCormack, W.M. (1991). HIV infection, genital ulcer disease, and crack cocaine use among patients attending a clinic for sexually transmitted diseases. *American Journal of Public Health*, 81, 1576-1579.

Christensen, D.N. (1983). Postmastectomy couple counseling: An outcome study of a structured treatment protocol. *Journal of Sex and Marital Therapy*, 9, 266-274.

Christensen–Szalanski, J.J.J. (1984). Discount functions and the measurement of patients' values: women's decisions during childbirth. *Medical Decision Making*, 4, 47-58.

Christopher, E. (1991). Family planning and reproductive decisions. *Journal of Reproductive and Infant Psychology*, 9, 217-226.

Chu, S.Y., Buehler, J.W. and Berkelman, R.L. (1990). Impact of the human immunodeficiency virus epidemic on mortality in women of reproductive ages, United States. *Journal of the American Medical Association*, 264, 225-229.

Chu, S.Y., Peterman, T.A., Doll, L.S., Buehler, J.W. and Curran, J.W. (1992). AIDS in bisexual men in the United States: Epidemiology and transmission to women. *American Journal of Public Health*, 82, 220-224.

Clarke, L. (1984). Psychosocial aspects of contraception. In A. Broome and L. Wallace (Eds.). *Psychology and gynaecological problems*, London: Tavistock.

Cleary, P.D., Van Devanter, N., Rogers, T.F., Singer, E., Shipton–Levy, R., Steilen, M. et al. (1991). Behavior changes after notification of HIV infection. *American Journal of Public Health*, 81, 1586-1590.

Cochrane, R. (1983). *The social creation of mental illness.* London: Longman. London.

Cochrane, R. (1988). Marriage, separation and divorce. In S. Fisher and J. Reason (Eds.). *Handbook of life stress, cognition and health*. Chichester: John Wiley.

Cochrane, R. and Sobol, M. (1980). Life stresses and psychological consequences. In M.P. Feldman and J. Orford (Eds.). *The social psychology of psychological problems*. Chichester: Wiley.

Cochrane, R. and Stopes-Roe, M. (1980). Factors affecting the distribution of psychological symptoms in urban areas of England. *Acta Psychiatrica Scandinavica*, 61, 445-460.

Cochrane, R. and Stopes-Roe, M. (1981). Women, marriage, employment and mental health. *British Journal of Psychiatry*, 139, 373-381.

Cochrane, R. (1983). *The social creation of mental illness.* London: Longman.

Cockburn, J., Murphy, B. and Schofield, P. (1991). Development of a strategy to encourage attendance for screening mammography. *Health Education Research*, 6, 279-290.

Cogan, R. and Spinnato, J.A. (1988). Social support during premature labor: effects on labor and the newborn. *Journal of Psychosomatic Obstetrics and Gynaecology*, 8, 209-216.

Cohen, S. and Syme, S.L. (1985). Issues in the study and application of social support. In S.

Cohen and S.L. Syme (Eds.), *Social support and health*, New York: Academic Press, 1985.

Colditz, G.A., Willett, W.C., Stampfer, M.J., Rosner, B., Speizer F.E. and Hennekens, C.H. (1987). Menopause and the risk of coronary heart disease in women. *New England Journal of Medicine*, **316**, 1105–1110.

Collins, A. and Frankenhauser, M. (1978). Stress responses in male and female engineering students. *Journal of Human Stress*, **4**, 43–48.

Connolly, K.J., Edelman, R.J. and Cooke, I.D. (1987). Distress and marital problems associated with infertility. *Journal of Reproductive and Infant Psychology*, **5**, 49–57.

Cooper, P.J., Campbell, E.A., Day, A. Kennerley, H. and Bond, A. (1988). Non-psychotic psychiatric disorder after childbirth: a prospective study of prevalence, incidence, course and nature. *British Journal of Psychiatry*, **152**, 799–806.

Cooper, P.J. and Fairburn, C.G. (1984). Cognitive behaviour therapy for anorexia nervosa: Some preliminary findings. *Journal of Psychosomatic Research*, **28(6)**, 493–499.

Cooper, P.J., Waterman, G.C. and Fairburn, C.G. (1984). Women with eating problems: A community survey. *British Journal of Clinical Psychology*, **23**, 45–52.

Cooper, P., Gath, D., Rose, N. and Fieldsend, R. (1982). Psychological sequalae to elective sterilisation in childless women: a prospective study. *British Medical Journal*, **284**, 461–464.

Cotton, P. (1991). Medicine's arsenal in battling 'Dominant Dozen', other AIDS-associated opportunistic infections. *Journal of the American Medical Association*, **266**, 1476–1481.

Crisp, A.H. (1984). The psychopathology of anorexia nervosa: getting the "heat" out of the system. In A.J. Stunkard and E. Stellar (Eds.), *Eating and its disorders*. New York: Raven Press.

Crook, J., Rideout, E. and Browne, G. (1984). The prevalence of pain complaints in a general population *Pain*, **18**, 299–314.

Dalton, K. (1984). *The premenstrual syndrome and progesterone therapy*, 2nd edn, London: Heinemann.

Davey Smith, G., Bartley, M. and Blane, D. (1990). The Black report on socioeconomic inequalities in health 10 years on. *British Medical Journal*, **301**, 373–377.

Davidson, A.R. and Jaccard, J.J. (1975). Population psychology: a new look at an old problem. *Journal of Personality and Social Psychology*, **31**, 1073–1082.

Davis, D.I., Berenson, D., Steinglass, P. and Davis, S. (1974) The adaptive consequences of drinking. *Psychiatry*, **37**, 209–215.

Davis, H. (1986). Effects of biofeedback and cognitive therapy on stress in patients with breast cancer. *Psychological Reports*, **59**, 967–974.

Dawson, K. and Singer, D. (1990). Should fertile people have access to in vitro fertilisation? *British Medical Journal*, **300**, 167–170.

de Haes, J.C.J.M., van Oostrom, M.A. and Welraart K. (1986). The effect of radical and conserving surgery on quality of life of early breast cancer patients. *European Journal of Surgical Oncology*, **12**, 337–342.

Dean, C. and Surtees, P.G. (1989). Do psychological factors predict survival in breast cancer. *Journal of Psychosomatic Research*, **33**, 561–569.

Dean, K. (1989). Self-care components of lifestyle: The importance of gender, attitudes and their social situations. *Social Science and Medicine*, **29**, 137–152.

Denenberg, R. (1990, December). Women and HIV–related conditions. *The Positive Woman*, **1**, 5–7.

Derogatis, L.R., Morrow, G.R., Fetting, J., Penman, D., Piasetsky, S., Schmale, A.M., Henricho, M. and Carnicke, C.L.M. (1983). The prevalence of psychiatric disorders among cancer patients. *Journal of the American Medical Association*, **249**, 751–757.

Des Jarlais, D.C., Friedman, S.R. and Woods, J.S. (1990). Intravenous drug use and AIDS. In D.G. Ostrow (Ed.), *Behavioral Aspects of AIDS*. New York: Plenum.

Des Jarlais, D.C. and Stepherson, B. (1991). History, ethics, and politics in AIDS prevention research. *American Journal of Public Health*, **81**, 1393–1394.

Devlen, J., Maguire, P., Phillips, P., Crowther, D. and Chambers, H. (1987). Psychological problems associated with diagnosis and treatment of lymphomas. I: Retrospective study and II: Prospective study. *British Medical Journal*, 295, 953–957.

Dick Read, G (1942). *Revelation of childbirth*. London: William Heinemann.

Doherty, W.L., Schrott, H.G., Metcalf, L. and Lasiello–Vallas, L. (1983). Effect of spouse support and health beliefs on medication adherence. *Journal of Family Practice*, 17, 837–841.

Duncan, I.D. (1992). *Guidelines for clinical practice and programme management NHS cervical screening programme*. Oxford: Oxford Regional Health Authority: Screening publications.

Eaker, E.A., Packard, B., Wenger, N.K., Clarkson, T.B. and Tyroler, H.A. (1987). Coronary heart disease in women: Reviewing the evidence, identifying the needs: A summary of the proceedings. Administrative report. Bethesda, MD: National Heart, Lung, and Blood Institute, National Institutes of Health, 1–48.

Edelman, R.J. and Golombok, S. (1989). Stress and reproductive failure. *Journal of Reproductive and Infant Psychology*, 7, 79–86.

Edens, J.L., Larkin, K.T. and Abel, J.L. (1992). The effect of social support and physical touch on cardiovascular reactions to mental stress. *Journal of Psychosomatic Research*, 36, 371–382.

Ehrenreich, B. and English, D. (1979). *For her own good: 150 years of the expert's advice to women*. London: Pluto Press.

El-Sadr, W. and Capps, L. (1992). The challenge of minority recruitment in clinical trials for AIDS. *Journal of the American Medical Association*, 267, 954–957.

Elbourne, D., Oakley, A. and Chalmers, I. (1990). Social and psychological support during pregnancy. In J. Chalmers, M. Enkin, and M. Keirse (Eds.), *Effective care in pregnancy and childbirth*. Oxford: Oxford University Press.

Ellerbrock, T., Bush, T., Chamberland, M. and Oxtoby, M. (1991). Epidemiology of women with AIDS in the United States, 1981 through 1990. *Journal of the American Medical Association*, 265, 2971–2975.

Elliot, S.A., Sanjack, M. and Leverton, T.J. (1988). Parents groups in pregnancy. In B.H. Gottlieb (Ed.), *Marshalling social support*, London: Sage.

Endicott, J. and Halbreich, U. (1982). Retrospective report of premenstrual depressive changes: Factors affecting confirmation by daily ratings. *Psychopharmacology Bulletin*, 18, 109–112.

European Collaborative Study. (1991). Children born to women with HIV-1 infection: Natural history and risk of transmission. *The Lancet*, 337, 253–260.

Eysenck, S. (1961). Personality and pain assessment in childbirth of married and unmarried mothers. *Journal of Mental Science*, 104, 417–430.

Farrant, W. (1980). Stress after amniocentesis for high serum alpha–feto–protein concentrations. *British Medical Journal*, 281, 452.

Fawzy, F.I., Cousins, N. Fawzy, N., Kemeny, M.E., Elashoff, R. and Morton, D. (1990a). A structured psychiatric intervention for cancer patients: I. Changes over time in methods of coping and affective disturbance. Archives of General Psychiatry, 47, 720–725.

Fawzy, F.I., Kemeny, M.E., Fawzy, N., Elashoff, R., Morton, D., Cousins, N. and Fahey, J.L. (1990b). A structured psychiatric intervention for cancer patients: II Changes over time in immunological measures. *Archives of General Psychiatry*, 47, 729–735.

Feine, J.S., Bushnell, M.C., Mirsch, D. and Duncan, G.H. (1991). Sex differences in the perception of noxious heat stimuli. *Pain*, 44, 255–262.

Feinmann, C. (1985). Pain relief by anti–depressants: possible modes of action. *Pain*, 23, 1–8.

Felson, D.T. (1989). Epidemiologic research in fibromyalgia *Journal of Rheumatology*, 16, 7–11.

Ferlic, M., Goldman, A. and Kennedy, B.J. (1979). Group counseling in adult patients with advanced cancer. *Cancer*, 45, 760–766.

Fischer, A.A. (1987). Pressure algometry over normal muscles. Standard values, validity and reproductibility of pressure threshold. *Pain*, 30, 115–126.

Fishbein, M. (1972). Towards an understanding of family planning behaviors. *Journal of Applied Social Psychology*, 2, 214–227.

Fishbein, M. and Azjen, I. (1975). *Belief, attitude, intention and behaviour: an introduction to theory and research.* Reading, Mass: Addison-Wesley.

Flanagan, D., Burnyeat, S., Wade, B., Clarke and H. and Marten, R. (1988). Evaluation of a syringe exchange scheme. *Proceedings of the Fourth International Conference on AIDS*, 4, 388.

Fontana, A.F., Kerns, R.D., Rosenberg, R.L. and Colonese, K.L. (1989). Support, stress, and recovery from coronary heart disease: A longitudinal causal model. *Health Psychology*, 8, 175–193.

Ford, M.J. (1986). Invited review–The Irritable Bowel Syndrome. *Journal of Psychosomatic Research*, 30, 399–410.

Forrest, P. (1986). *Breast cancer screening.* Report to the Health Ministers of England, Wales, Scotland and Northern Ireland. London: HMSO.

Fox, B.H. (1978). Premorbid psychological factors as related to cancer incidence. *Journal of Behavioral Medicine*, 1, 45–133.

Fox, A.J. and Goldblatt, P.D. (1982). *OPCS Longitudinal study: Socio*-demographic mortality differentials 1971–75. London: HMSO

Fox, H.E. (1991). Obstetric issues and counselling women and parents. In P.A. Pizzo and C.M. Wilfert (Eds.), *Pediatric AIDS*. Baltimore, MD: Williams & Wilkins.

Fox, J. (1989) (Ed.), *Health inequalities in European countries*. Aldershot: Gower Publishing Co.

Frank, K. (1990). *Emily Brontë: A chainless soul.* London: Hamish Hamilton.

Frankenhaeuser, M., Lundberg, U. and Fredrikson, M. (1989). Stress on and off the job as related to sex and occupational status in white-collar workers. *Journal of Organizational Behavior*, 10, 321–346.

Frankenhaeuser, M. (1983). The sympathetic-adrenal and pituitary-adrenal response to challenge: Comparison between the sexes. In T.M. Dembroski, T.H. Schmidt and G. Blumchen (Eds.), *Biobehavioral bases of coronary heart disease*. Basel: Karger.

Fraser, I. (1986). How acceptable are menstrual disturbances to hormonal contraceptive users? In L. Dennerstein and I. Fraser (Eds.), *hormones and behaviour* The Netherlands: Elsevier.

French, K., Porter, A.M.D., Robinson, S.E. McCallum, F.R., Howie, J.G.R. and Roberts, M.M.(1982). Attendance at a breast screening clinic: A problem of administration or attitudes. *British Medical Journal*, 285, 617–620.

Freedman, R.R., Sabharwal, S.C. and Desai, N. (1987). Sex differences in peripheral vascular adrenergic receptors. *Circulation Research*, 61, 581–585.

Freeman, E.W., Sondheimer, S., Weinbaum, P.J. and Rickels, K. (1985). Evaluating pre-menstrual symptoms in medical practice. *Obstetrics and Gynecology*, 65, 500–505.

Friedman, M., Thoresen, C.E., Gill, J.J., Ulmer, D., Powell, L.H., Price, V.A., Brown, B., Thompson, L., Rabin, D., Breall, W.S., Bourg, E., Levy, R. and Dixon, T. (1986). Alteration of Type A behaviour and its effects on cardiac recurrences in postmyocardial infarction patients: Summary of the Recurrent Coronary Prevention Project. *American Heart Journal*, 112, 653–665.

Friedman, M., Thoresen, C.E., Gill, J.J., Powell, L.H., Ulmer, D., Thompson, L., Price, V.A., Rabin, D.D., Breal, W.S., Dixon, T., Levy, R.A. and Bourg, E. (1984). Alteration of Type A behavior and reduction in cardiac recurrences in post myocardial infarction patients. *American Heart Journal*, 108, 237–248.

Froberg, D., Gjerdingen, D. and Preston, M. (1986). Multiple roles and women's mental and physical health: what have we learned? *Women and Health*, 11, 79–96.

Fulton, J.P., Buechner, J.S., Scott, H.D. et al (1991). A study guided by the Health Belief Model of the predictors of breast cancer screening of women aged 40 and over. *Public Health Report*, 106, 410–420.

Funch, D.P. and Marshall, J. (1983). The role of stress, social support and function. *Psychosomatic Medicine*, 49, 13–34.

Garner, D.M. and Garfinkel, P.E. (1980). Socio-cultural factors in the development of anorexia nervosa. *Psychological Medicine*, 10, 647–656.

Gater, R.A., Dean, C. and Morris, J. (1989). The contribution of childbearing to the sex difference in first admission rates for affective psychosis. *Psychological Medicine*, 19, 719-724.

Gerin, W., Pieper, C., Levy, R. and Pickering, T.G. (1992). Social support in social interaction: A moderator of cardiovascular reactivity. *Psychosomatic Medicine*, 54, 324-336.

Girdler, S.S., Pedersen, C.A., Stern, R.A. and Light, K.C. (in press). The menstrual cycle and premenstrual syndrome: Modifiers of cardiovascular reactivity in women. *Health Psychology*.

Girdler, S.S., Turner, J.R., Sherwood, A. and Light, K.C. (1990). Gender differences in blood pressure control during a variety of behavioral stressors. *Psychosomatic Medicine*, 52, 571-591.

Gladwell, M. (1992, February 1). FDA panel recommends approval of female condom. *The Washington Post*, Section A, p. a01.

Glanz, K. and Lerman, C. (in press). Psychosocial impact of breast cancer: A critical review. *Annals of Behavioral Medicine*.

Goetsch, V.L., Burnette, M.M., Weiner, A.L., Koehn, J.A., Vanin, J. and Clements, J-N. (1991). An investigation of the influence of expectancies on affective and physical changes associated with oral contraceptive use. *Journal of Psychosomatic Obstetrics and Gynaecology*, 12, 209-216.

Gold, E.R. (1986). Long term effects of sexual victimization in childhood: an attributional approach. *Journal of Consulting and Clinical Psychology*, 54, 471-475.

Goldberg, D. and Huxley, P. (1980). *Mental illness in the community*, London: Tavistock.

Goolkasian, P. (1985). Phase and sex effects in pain perception: A critical review. *Psychology of Women Quarterly*, 9, 15-28.

Gottesman, D. and Lewis, M. (1982). Differences in crisis reactions among cancer and surgery patients. *Journal of Consulting and Clinical Psychology*, 50, 381-388.

Gove, W.R. (1972). The relationship between sex roles, marital status, and mental illness. *Social Forces*, 51, 34-44.

Gove, W.R. (1984). Gender differences in mental and physical illness: the effects of fixed roles and nurturant roles. *Social Science and Medicine*, 19, 77-83.

Gove, W.R. and Tudor, J.F. (1973). Adult sex roles and mental illness. *American Journal of Sociology*, 78, 812-835.

Graham, C.A. and Sherwin, B.B. (1992). A prospective treatment study of premenstrual symptoms using a triphasic oral contraceptive. *Journal of Psychosomatic Research*, 36, 1-10.

Green, J. (1990a). Is the baby alright and other worries. *Journal of Reproductive and Infant Psychology*, 8, 225-226.

Green, J.M. (1990b). Who is unhappy after childbirth?: Antenatal and intrapartum correlates from a prospective study. *Journal of Reproductive and Infant Psychology*, 8, 225-226.

Greenwald, P. and Cullen, J.W. (1985). The new emphasis in cancer control. *Journal of the National Cancer Institute*, 74, 543-551.

Gritz, E.R. (1991). Biobehavioral factors in smoking and smoking cessation. Paper presented at the National Heart, Lung and Blood Institute Conference on Women, Behavior and Cardiovascular Disease, Chevy Chase, MD, September 25-27, 1991.

Gritz, E.R., Klesges, R.C. and Meyers, A.W. (1989). Smoking and body weight: Implications for interventions and post-cessation weight control. *Annals of Behavioral Medicine*, 11, 144-153.

Guillebaud, J. (1991a). *The pill*. Oxford: Oxford University Press.

Guillebaud, J. (1991b). Contraception after pregnancy. *The British Journal of Family Planning*, 16 (suppl.). 16-19.

Guinan, M.E. and Hardy, A. (1987a). Epidemiology of AIDS in women in the United States: 1981 through 1986. *Journal of the American Medical Association*, 257, 2039-2042.

Guinan, M.E. and Hardy, A. (1987b). Women and AIDS: The future is grim. *Journal of the American Women's Medical Association*, 42, 157-158.

Gull, W.W. (1874). Anorexia nervosa (aspepsia hysterica, anorexia hysterica). *Transactions of* the Clinical Society, 7, 22–28.

Gwinn, M., Pappaioanu, M., George, J.R., Hannon, W.H., Wasser, S.C., Redus, M.A. *et al.* (1991). Prevalence of HIV infection in childbearing women in the United States. *Journal of the American Medical Association*, 265, 1704–1708.

Haavio-Mannila, E. (1986). Inequalities in health and gender. *Social Science and Medicine*, 22, 141–149.

Hakama, M. (1982). Trends in cancer incidence. In K. Magnus (Ed.). Washington: Hemisphere.

Halbreich, U. and Endicott, J. (1985). Methodological issues in studies of premenstrual changes. *Psychoneuroendocrinology*, 10, 15–33.

Hardy, J.D., Wolff, H.G. and Goodell, H. (1967). *Pain sensations and reactions*. New York: Hafner.

Harkness, J. and Gijsbers, K. (1989). Pain and stress during childbirth and time of day. *Ethology and Sociobiology*, 10, 255–261.

Hart, N. (1989). Sex differentials and mortality in Europe. In J. Fox (Ed.), *Health inequalities in Europe*. Aldershot: Gower Publishing Co.

Hart, W.G., Coleman, G.J. and Russell, J.W. (1987). Assessment of premenstrual symptomatology: A re-evaluation of the predictive validity of self-report. *Journal of Psychosomatic Research*, 31, 185–190.

Haskett, R.F., Steiner, M., Osmun, J.N. and Carroll, B.J. (1980). Severe premenstrual tension: Delineation of the syndrome. *Biological Psychiatry*, 15, 121–139.

Hazuda, P.H., Haffner, S.M., Stern, M.P., Knapp, J.A., Eiffer, C.W. and Rosenthal, M. (1986). Employment status and women's protection against coronary heart disease. *American Journal of Epidemiology*, 123, 623–640.

Healy, B. (1991). The Yentl Syndrome. *New England Journal of Medicine*, 325, 274–276.

Helsing, K., Szklo, M. and Comstock, G. (1981). Factors associated with mortality after widowhood. *American Journal of Public Health*, 71, 802–809.

Herman, C.P. (1978). Restrained eating. *Psychiatric Clinics of North America*, 1(3), 593–607.

Herman, C.P. and Polivy, J. (1980). Restrained eating. In A. Stunkard (Ed.), *Obesity*. Philadelphia: Saunders.

Herman, C.P., Polivy, J. and Silver, R. (1979). Effects of an observer on eating behavior: The induction of sensible eating. *Journal of Personality*, 47(1), 85–99.

Herzberg, B.N., Draper, K.C., Johnson, A.I. and Nicol, C.C. (1971). Oral contraceptives, depression and libido. *British Medical Journal*, 3, 495–500.

Higgins, M.W. (1990). Women and coronary heart disease. Then and now. *Women's Health Issues*, 1, 5–11.

Higgins, M.W. (1984). Changing patterns of smoking and risk of disease. In E.B. Gold (Ed.), *The changing risk of disease in women: An epidemiologic approach*. Lexington, MA: Collagomre.

Hiller, C.A. and Slade, P. (1989). The impact of antenatal classes on knowledge, anxiety and confidence in primiparous. *Journal of Reproductive and Infant Psychology*, 7, 3–15.

Hobbs, P., Elkind, A., Haran, D. Eardley, A., Spencer, B., Pendleton, L.L. and Chisholm, D.K. (1985). Screening for cervical cancer: An opportunity for change. In A. Smith (Ed.) *Recent advances in community medicine*, Edinburgh; New York: Churchill Livingstone.

Holden, J.A., Sagovsky, R.S. and Cox, J.L. (1989). Counselling in a general practice setting: a controlled trial of health visitor intervention in postnatal depression. *British Medical Journal*, 298, 233–6.

Holland, W.W. and Stewart, S. (1990). *Screening in health care – benefit or bane?* London: Nuffield Provincial Hospital Trust.

Hopkins, J., Marcus, M. and Campbell, S.B. (1984). Postpartum depression: a critical review. *Psychological Bulletin*, 95, 498–515.

House, J.S., McMichael, A.J., Wells, J.A., Kaplan, B.H. and Landerman, L.R. (1979). Occupational stress and health among factory workers. *Journal of Health and Social Behavior*,

20, 139–160.

House, J.S., Robbins, C. and Metzner, H.L. (1982). The association of social relationships and activities to mortality: Prospective evidence from Tecumseh Community Health Study. *American Journal of Epidemiology*, 116, 123–140.

Houts, P.S., Whitney, C.W., Mortel, R. and Bartholomew, M.J. (1986). Former cancer patients as counselors of newly diagnosed cancer patients. *Journal of the National Cancer Institute*, 76, 793–796.

Hughson, A.V.M., Cooper, A.F., McArdle, C.S. and Smith, D.C. (1987). Psychosocial effects of radiotherapy after mastectomy. *British Medical Journal*, 294, 1515–1518.

Hunt, S.M., Alexander, F. and Robert, M.M. (1988). Attenders and non attenders at a breast screening clinic: A comparative study. *Public Health*, 102, 3–10.

Hunt, K. (1990). The first pill taking generation: past and present use of contraception among a cohort of women born in the early 50's. *The British Journal of Family Planning*, 16, 3–15.

Hunt, K. and Allandale, E. (1990). Predicting contraceptive method usage among women in West Scotland. *Journal of Biosocial Science*, 22, 405–421.

Hunter, M. (1989). Gynaecology. In A. Broome (ed.), *Health psychology*, Broome, A. London: Chapman and Hall.

Hypertension Detection and Follow-up Program Cooperative Group (1979). Five-year findings of the hypertension detection and follow-up program. II. Mortality by race, sex and age. *Journal of the American Medical Association*, 242, 2572–2577.

International Agency for Research in Cancer: Working Group on Evaluation of Cervical Cancer Programmes (1986). Screening for squamous cervical cancer. *British Medical Journal*, 293, 659–64.

Istvan, J. (1986). Stress, anxiety, and birth outcomes: a critical review of the evidence. *Psychological Bulletin*, 4, 110–111.

Jahoda, M. and Rush, H. (1980). Work, employment and unemployment: An overview of ideas and research results in the social science literature. Science Policy Unit, Occasional Paper Series No. 12.

James, F.R., Large, R.G., Bushnell, J.A. and Wells, J.E. (1991). Epidemiology of pain in New Zealand. *Pain*, 44, 279–283.

Jeffery, R.W. (1991). Behavioral influences on diet, obesity and weight control strategies in women. Paper presented at the National Heart, Lung and Blood Institute Conference on Women, Behavior and Cardiovascular Disease, Chevy Chase, MD, September 25–27, 1991.

Johnson, J.V. (1986). The impact of workplace social support and work control upon cardiovascular disease in Sweden. Division of Environmental and Organizational Psychology Research Report No. 1. University of Stockholm.

Johnson, R.W., Ostrow, D.G. and Joseph, J. (1990). Educational strategies for prevention of sexual transmission of HIV. In D.G. Ostrow, (Ed.), *Behavioral aspects of AIDS*. New York: Plenum

Johnson, C., Lewis, C., Love, S., Stuckey, M. and Lewis, L. (1983). A descriptive survey of dieting and bulimic behaviour in a female high-school population. *Journal of Youth and Adolescence*, 13, 15–26.

Johnston, M., Shaw, R.W. and Bird, D. (1987). "Test-tube baby" procedures: stress and judgements under uncertainty. *Psychology and Health*, 1, 25–38.

Johnston, M., Shaw, P., Shaw, R.W. and Adib, T. (1990). Optimism about success in IVF. *Journal of Reproductive and Infant Psychology*, 8, 212.

Kandel, D.B., Davies, M. and Ravies, V.H. (1985). The stressfulness of daily social roles for women: marital, occupational and household roles. *Journal of Health and Social Behaviour*, 26, 64–66.

Kannel, W.B. (1977). Importance of hypertension as a major risk factor in cardiovascular disease. In J. Genest, E. Koiw and O. Kuchel (Eds.), *Hypertension: Physiopathology and treatment*. New York, McGraw-Hill.

Kaplan, R.M., Anderson, J.P. and Wingard, D.L. (1991). Gender differences in health–related quality of life. *Health Psychology*, 10, 86–93.

Kaplan, R.M., Atkins, C.J. and Lenhand, L. (1982). Coping with a stressful sigmoidoscopy. Evaluation of cognitive and relaxation preparations. *Journal of Behavioral Medicine*, 5, 67–82.

Kaplan, J.R., Manuck, S.B., Clarkson, T.B., Lusso, F.M. and Taub, D.M. (1982). Social status, environment and atherosclerosis in cynomolgus monkeys. *Arteriosclerosis*, 2, 359–368.

Karpf, A. (1988). *Doctoring the media: The reporting of health and medicine*. New York: Routledge.

Kehrer, B.H. and Wolin, C.M. (1979). Impact of income maintenance on low birthweight. *Journal of Human Resources*, 14, 434–462.

Kessler, R.C., McLeod, J.D., and Wethington, E. (1985). The costs of caring: A perspective on the relationship between sex and psychological distress. In I.G. Sarason and B.R. Sarson (Eds.), *Social support: Theory, research and applications*. Boston: Martinus Nijhoff.

Kiecolt–Glaser, J.K., Glaser, R., Strain, E., Stout, J., Tarr, K., Holliday, J. and Speicher, C. (1986). Modulation of cellular immunity in medical students. *Journal of Behavioral Medicine*, 9, 5–21.

Kiecolt–Glaser, J.K., Fisher, L.D., Ogrocki, P., Stout, J.C., Speicher, C.E. and Glaser, R. (1987). Marital quality, marital disruption, and immune function. Psychosomatic Medicine, 49, 13–34.

King, J. (1984). The Health Belief Model. *Nursing Times* October 24, 53–55.

King, A. (1991). Biobehavioral variables, exercise and cardiovascular disease in women. Paper presented at the National Heart, Lung and Blood Institute Conference on Women, Behavior and Cardiovascular Disease, Chevy Chase, MD, September 25–27, 1991.

King, K.B., Nail, L.M., Kreamer, K., Strohl, R.A. and Johnson, J.E. (1985). Patients' descriptions of the experience of receiving radiation therapy. *Oncology Nursing Forum*, 12, 55–61.

Kitzinger, S. (1962). *The experience of childbirth*. London: Golancz.

Kitzinger, S. (1989). Perceptions of pain in home and hospital deliveries. In E.V. van Hall and W. Everaerd (Eds.). *The free woman: Women's health in the 1990s*. Lancashire: the Parthenon Publishing Company Limited.

Klaus, M.H., Kennel, J.H., Robertson, S.S. and Sosa, R. (1986). Effects of social support during parturition on material and infant morbidity. *British Medical Journal*, 293, 585–587.

Koonin, L.M., Ellerbrock, T.V., Atrash, H.K., Roger, M.F., Smith, J.C., Hogue, C.J.R. *et al.* (1989). Pregnancy–associated deaths due to AIDS in the United States. *Journal of the American Medical Association*, 261, 1306–1309.

Kotelchuck, M., Schwartz, J.B., Anderka, M.T. and Finison, K.S. (1984). WIC participation and pregnancy outcomes: Massachusetts statewide evaluation project. *American Journal of Public Health*, 74, 1086–1092.

Krantz, D.S. and Manuck, S.B. (1984). Acute psychophysiologic reactivity and risk of cardiovascular disease: A review and methodologic critique. *Psychological Bulletin*, 96, 435–464.

Labs, S.M. and Wurtele, S.K. (1986). Fetal Health Locus of Control Scale: Development and validation. *Journal of Consulting Clinical Psychology*, 54, 814–819.

LaCroix, A–Z. and Haynes, S.G. (1987). Gender differences in the health effects of workplace roles. In R.C. Barnett, L. Biener and G.K. Baruch (Eds.), *Gender and stress*. New York: Free Press.

Lambers, K.J., Trimbos–Kemper, G.C.M. and van Hall, E.V. (1984). Regret and reversal of sterilization. In Broome, A. (Ed.), *Health psychology*, London: Chapman and Hall.

Lanksy, S.B., List, M.A., Herrmann, C.A., Ets–Hokin, E.G., DasGupta, T.K., Wilbanks, G.D. and Hendrickson, F.R. (1985). Absence of major depressive disorders in female cancer patients. *Journal of Clinical Oncology*, 3, 1553–1560.

Lasegue, Dr. (1873). On hysterical anorexia. *Medical Times and Gazette*, 265–266 (6 Sept) &

367–369 (27 Sept). (From: Archives Generales de Medecine, April 1873).

Lawrence, M. (1984). *The Anorexic Experience*. London: Women's Press.

Lawson, S., Cole, R.A. and Templeton, A.A. (1979). The effects of laparascopic sterilisation by diathermy or silastic bands on post operative pain, menstrual symptoms and sexuality. *British Journal of Obstetrics and Gynaecology*, **86**, 659–663.

Lazarus, R.S. and Folkman, S. (1984). *Stress appraisal and coping*. New York: Springer.

Lazarus, R.S., Opton, E.M., Jr., Nomikos, M.S. and Rankin, N.O. (1965). The principle of short–circuiting of threat: Further evidence. *Journal of Personality*, **33**, 622–635.

Lederman, R.P., Lederman, E., Work, B.A. and McCann, D.S. (1978). The relationship of maternal anxiety, plasma catecholamines and plasma cortisol to progress in labour. *American Journal of Obstetrics and Gynecology*, **132**, 495–500.

Leon, G.R. (1980). Is it bad not to be thin? *American Journal of Clinical Nutrition*, **33**, 174–175.

Lerner, D.J. and Kannel, W.B. (1986). Patterns of coronary heart disease morbidity and mortality in the sexes: A 26–year follow–up of the Framingham population. *American Heart Journal*, **111**, 383–390.

Leviathan, U. and Cohen, J. (1985). Gender differences in life expectancy among kibbutz members. *Social Science and Medicine*, **21**, 545–551.

Levin, P.M., Silberfarb, P.M. and Lipowski, Z.J. (1978). Mental disorders in cancer patients: A study of 100 psychiatric referrals. *Cancer*, **42**, 1385–1391.

Levine, F.M. and De Simone, L.L. (1991). The effects of experimenter gender on pain report in male and female subjects. *Pain*, **44**, 69–72.

Levine, C. and Dubler, N.N. (1990). Uncertain risks and bitter realities: The reproductive choices of HIV–infected women. *The Millbank Quarterly*, **68**, 321–351.

Levinson, G. and Schnider, S.M. (1979). Catecholamines: the effects of maternal fear and its treatment on uterine function and circulation. *Birth and Family Journal*, **6**, 167–174.

Lewis, C. (1986). *Becoming a father*. Milton Keynes: Open University Press.

Lewis, V.J. and Booth, D.A. (1986). Causal influences within an individual's dieting thoughts, feelings and behaviour. In J.M. Diehl and C. Leitzmann (Eds.), *Measurement and determinants of food habits*. Wageningen: University Department of Human Nutrition.

Lewis, V.J. and Blair, A.J. (1991). The social context of eating disorders. In: Cochrane, R. and Carroll, D. (Eds.), *Psychology and Social Issues: A Tutorial Text*. London: Falmer Press.

Lewis, V.J., Blair, A.J. and Booth, D.A. (1992). Outcome of group therapy for body–image emotionality and weight–control self–efficacy. *Behavioural Psychotherapy*, **20**, 155–165.

Ley, P. (1988). *Communicating with patients*. London: Croom Helm.

Lichtman, R.R. and Taylor, S.E. (1986). Close relationships and the female cancer patient. In B.L. Andersen (Ed.), *Women with cancer: Psychological perspectives*. New York: Springer–Verlag.

Liebeskind, J.C. and Paul, L.A. (1977). Psychological and physiological mechanisms of pain. *Annual Review of Psychology*, **28**, 41–60.

Light, E. and Lebowitz, B. (1988) (Eds.), *Alzheimer's disease treatment and family stress: Directions for research*. Washington, C.D.: National Institute of Mental Health.

Light, K.C., Dolan, C.A., Davis, M.R. and Sherwood, A. (1992). Cardiovascular responses to an active coping challenge as predictors of blood pressure patterns 10 to 15 years later. *Psychosomatic Medicine*, **54**, 217–230.

Light, K.C., Turner, J.R., Hinderliter, A.L. and Sherwood, A. (in press). Race and gender comparisons: I. Hemodynamic responses to a series of stressors. *Health Psychology*.

Lindemann, C. (1977). Factors affecting the use of contraceptives in the non marital context. In R. Gemme and C.C. Wheeler, (Eds.), *Progress in sexology*, New York: Plenum.

Lipid Metabolism Branch, Division of Heart and Vascular Diseases, National Heart, Lung and Blood Institute (1980). The Lipid Research Clinics population studies data book. Vol. 1. The prevalence study: Aggregate distributions of lipids, lipoproteins and selected variables in 11 North American populations. Bethesda, MD, National Institute of Health (NIH Publication

No. 80–1527).

Lobo, R.A. (1990). Estrogen and cardiovascular disease. *Annals of the New York Academy of Sciences*, **592**, 286–294.

Logue, C.M. and Moos, R.H. (1986). Perimenstrual symptoms: Prevalence and risk factors. *Psychosomatic Medicine*, **48**, 388–414.

Low, N.K. (1989). Explaining the pain of active labor: The importance of maternal confidence. *Research in Nursing and Health*, **12**, 237–245.

Low, M.R. (1984). Dietary concern, weight fluctuation and weight status: Further explorations of the restraint scale. *Behaviour Research and Therapy*, **22**, 243–248.

Luker, K. (1975). *Taking chances: abortion and the decision not to contracept*. Berkely, California: University of California Press.

Lundberg, U., de Chateau, P., Winberg, J. and Frankenhaeuses, M. (1981). Catecholaminic and cortisol excretion patterns in three year old children and their parents. *Journal of Human Stress*, **7**, 3–11.

Lyketsos, G., Arapakis, G., Psaras, M., Photiou, I., and Blackburn, I.M. (1982). Psychological characteristics of hypertensive and ulcer patients. *Journal of Psychosomatic Research*, **26**, 255–262.

MacGregor, J.E., Moss, S.M., Parkin, D.M. and Day, N.E. (1985). A case control study of cervical cancer screening in North-East Scotland. *British Medical Journal*, **290**, 1543–1546.

Macintyre, S. (1986). The patterning of health by social position in contemporary Britain: Directions for sociological research. *Science and Medicine*, **23**, 393–415.

MacLean, A., Sinfield, D., Klein, S. and Harden, B. (1984). Women who decline breast screening. *Journal of Epidemiology and Community Health*, **38**, 278–283.

Magni, G., Caldieron, C., Rigatti–Luchini, S. and Merskey, H. (1990). Depression and pain. *Pain*, **43**, 299–307.

Macgregor, J.E., Moss, S.M. Parkin, D.M. and Day, N.E. (1985). A case control study of cervical cancer screening in North-East Scotland. *British Medical Journal*, **290**, 1543–1546.

Maguire, G.P., Lee, E.G., Bevington, D.J., Kuchemann, C.S., Crabtree, R.J. and Cornell, C.E. (1978). Psychiatric problems in the first year after mastectomy. *British Medical Journal*, **1**, 963–965.

Maguire, P., Hopwood, P., Tarrier, N. and Howell, T. (1985). Treatment of depression in cancer patients. *Acta Psychiatrica Scandinavia*, **72** (suppl. 320), 81–84.

Malone, M.D. and Strube, M.J. (1988). Meta–analysis of non–medical treatments for chronic pain. *Pain*, **34**, 231–244.

Management Committee (1980). The Australian therapeutic trial in mild hypertension: Report by the Management Committee. *The Lancet*, **1**, 1261–1267.

Management Committee of the Australian Therapeutic Trial of Mild Hypertension (1981). Treatment of mild hypertension in the elderly. *Medical Journal of Australia*, **2**, 398–402.

Manuel, G.M., Roth, S., Keefe, F.J. and Brantley, B.A. (1987, Winter). Coping with cancer. *Journal of Human Stress*, 149–158.

Marin, B.V., Marin, G. and Juarez, R. (1988). Strategies for enhancing the cultural appropriateness of AIDS prevention campaigns. Paper presented at the 68th Annual Convention of the Western Psychological Association, Burlingame, CA, April 28–May 1.

Marks, G., Richardson, J.L. and Maldonado, N. (1991). Self disclosure of HIV infection to sexual partners. *American Journal of Public Health*, **81**, 1321–1323.

Marmot, M.G. and Davey Smith, G. (1989). Why are the Japanese living longer? *British Medical Journal*, **299**, 1547–1551.

Marmot, M.G., Shipley, M.J. and Rose, G. (1984). Inequalities in health – specific explanations of a general pattern? *The Lancet*, **1**, 1003–1006.

Marteau, T.M., Johnston, M., Kidd, J., Michie, S., Cook, R., Slack, J. and Shaw, R.W. (1992). Psychological models in predicting uptake of prenatal screening. *Psychology and Health*, **6**,

13–22.

Masters, W.H. and Johnson, V.E. (1966). *Human sexual response*. Boston: Little Brown and Co.

Matarazzo, J.D. (1980). Behavioral health and behavioral medicine: Frontiers of a new health psychology. *American Psychologist*, 35, 807–817.

Matthews, K.A. (1989). Are sociodemographic variables markers for psychological determinants of health. *Health Psychology*, 8, 641–648.

Matthews, K.A., Davis, M.C., Stoney, C.M., Owens, J.F. and Caggiula, A.R. (1991). Does the gender relevance of the stressor influence sex differences in psychophysiological responses? *Health Psychology*, 10, 112–120.

Matthews, K.A. (1989). Interactive effects of behavior and reproductive hormones on sex differences in risk for coronary heart disease. *Health Psychology*, 8, 373–387.

Matthews, K.A. and Stoney, C.M. (1988). Influence of sex and age on cardiovascular responses during stress. *Psychosomatic Medicine*, 50, 46–56.

Mayer, J.A. and Solomon, L.J. (in press). Breast self-examination skill and frequency: A review. *Annals of Behavioral Medicine*.

Mays, V.M. and Cochran, S.D. (1988). Issues in the perception of AIDS risk and risk reduction activities by Black and Hispanic/Latina women. *American Psychologist*, 43, 949–957.

McGill, H.C., Jr. and Stern, M.P. (1979). Sex and atherosclerosis. In R. Papletti, A.M. Gotto, Jr. (Eds.), *Atherosclerosis Reviews*. New York: Raven Press.

McGrath, E., Veita, G.P., Strickland, B.R. and Russo, N.F. (1990) *Women and depression: risk factors and treatment issues*, Washington, D.C.: American Psychological Association.

McIlwaine, G.M. (1989). Women and domestic violence. *British Medical Journal*, 299, 995–996.

McIlwaine, G.M., Rowarth, M. and Wallace, A.M. (1992). Users views. Report of the Acceptibility Committee of the Scottish Breast Screening Service.

Mechanic, D. (1982). The epidemiology of illness behaviour and its relationship to physical and psychological distress. In D. Mechanic (Ed.), *Symptoms, illness*–behavior and help–seeking. New York: Prodist.

Medical Research Council Working Party. (1985). MRC trial of mild hypertension: Principal results. *British Medical Journal*, 291, 197–204.

Melzack, R. (1984). The myth of painless childbirth (the John J. Bonica lecture). *Pain*, 19, 321–337.

Melzack, R. and Wall, P. (1991). *The challenge of pain*. New York: Penguin Books.

Menkes, M.S., Matthews, K.A., Krantz, D.S., Lundberg, V., Mead, L.A., Qaqish, B., Liang, K.-Y., Thomas, C.B. and Pearson, T.A. (1989). Cardiovascular reactivity to the cold pressor test as a predictor of hypertension. *Hypertension*, 14, 524–530.

Merikangas, K.R., Weissman, M.M. and Pauls, D.L. (1985). Genetic factors in the sex ratio of major depression. *Psychological Medicine*, 15, 63–70.

Metcalf, M.G. and Hudson, S.M. (1985). The premenstrual syndrome: Selection of women for treatment trials. *Journal of Psychosomatic Research*, 29, 631–638.

Metcalf, M.G., Livesey, J.H., Well, J.E., Braiden, V., Hudson, S.M. and Bamber, L. (1991). Premenstrual syndrome in hysterectomized women; mood and symptom cyclicity. *Journal of Psychosomatic Research*, 35, 555–567.

Metson, D. (1988). Lessons from an audit of unplanned pregnancies. *British Medical Journal*, 904–906.

Metson, D., Kaassianos, G., Norman, D.P. and Moriarty, J.M.A. (1991). Effect of information leaflets on long term recall: Useful or useless? *The British Journal of Family Planning*, 17, 21–23.

Meyerowitz, B.E., Watkins, I.K. and Sparks, F.C. (1983). Psychosocial implications of adjuvant chemotherapy. A two year followup. *Cancer*, 1541–1545.

Michie, S., Marteau, T.M. and Kidd, J. (1990). Cognitive predictors of attendance at antenatal classes. *British Journal of Clinical Psychology*, 57, 1059–1068.

Miles, A. (1988). *Women and mental illness*. Brighton: Wheatshead.

Miles, A. (1991). *Women, health and medicine*. Milton Keynes: Open University Press.

Miles (1991). *Women, health and medicine*. Milton Keynes: Open University Press.

Miller, H.G., Turner, C.F. and Moses, L.E. (1990). *AIDS: The second decade*. Washington, DC: National Academy Press.

Minkoff, H.L. (1987). Care of pregnant women infected with human immunodeficiency virus. *Journal of the American Medical Association*, **258**, 2714.

Minkoff, H.L. and DeHovitz, J.A. (1991). Care of women infected with the human immuno–deficiency virus. *Journal of the American Medical Association*, **266**, 2253–2257.

Minkoff, H.L. and Feinkind, L. (1989). Management of pregnancies of HIV–infected women. *Clinical Obstetrics and Gynecology*, **32**, 467–476.

Minkoff, H.L. and Landesman, S.H. (1988). The case for routinely offering prenatal testing for human immunodeficiency virus. *American Journal of Obstetrics and Gynecology*, **159**, 793–796.

Minkoff, H.L. and Moreno, J.D. (1990). Drug prophylaxis for human immunodeficiency virus–infected pregnant women: Ethical considerations. *American Journal of Obstetrics and Gynecology*, **163**, 1111–1114.

Mira, M., Vizzard, J. and Abraham, S.F. (1985). Personality characteristics in the menstrual cycle. *Journal of Psychosomatic Obstetrics and Gynecology*, **4**, 329–334.

Mira, M., McNeil, D., Fraser, I.S., Vizzard, J. and Abraham, S. (1986). Mefenamic acid in the treatment of premenstrual syndrome. *Obstetrics and Gynecology*, **68**, 395–398.

Mirsky, I.A. (1958). Physiologic, psychologic, and social determinants in the etiology of duodenal ulcer. *American Journal of Digestive Diseases*, **3**, 285–314.

Mitchell, J.L. and Heagarty, M. (1991). Special considerations of minorities. In P.A. Pizzo and C.M. Wilfert (Eds.), *Pediatric AIDS*. Baltimore, MD: Williams & Wilkins.

Morris, T., Greer, H.S. and White, P. (1977). Psychological and social adjustment to mastectomy: A two–year follow–up study. *Cancer*, **40**, 2381–2387.

Morse, C.A. and Dennerstein, L. (1988). Cognitive therapy for premenstrual syndrome. In M.G. Brush and E.M. Goudsmit (Eds.), *Functional disorders of the menstrual cycle*. Chichester: Wiley.

Moser, K.A. and Goldbalt, P.O. (1985). Mortality of women in the OPCS Longitudinal Study: Differentials by own occupation and household and housing characteristics. Social Statistics Research Unit Working Paper No. 26. London: City University.

Muldoon, M.F., Manuck, S.B. and Matthews, K.A. (1990). Lowering cholesterol concentrations and mortality: A quantitative review of primary prevention trials. *British Medical Journal*, **301**, 309–314.

Nakajima, G.A. and Rubin, H.C. (1991). Lack of racial, gender, and behavior-risk diversity in psychiatric research on AIDS/HIV in the United States. *Proceedings of the Seventh International Conference on AIDS*, **7**, 193.

National Center for Health Statistics. (1989). Publication No. PHS, 89–1232. Washington: U.S. Government Printing Office.

National Institute of Allergy and Infectious Disease, Centers for Disease Control. (1991, August). U.S. Public Health Service National Conference: Women and HIV Infection. *Clinical Courier*, 1–8.

Neilson, J. and Grant, A.J. (1990). Ultrasound in pregnancy. In J. Chalmers, M. Enkin, M. Keirse (Eds.), *Effective care in pregnancy and childbirth*, Oxford: Oxford University Press.

Neuling, S.J. and Winefield, H.R. (1988). Social support and recovery after surgery for breast cancer: Frequency and correlates of supportive behaviors by family, friends, and surgeon. *Social Science and Medicine*, **27**, 385–392.

Newsweek. (1991, December 9). Safer sex. pp. 52–56.

Newton, R.W. (1988). Psychological aspects of pregnancy: the scope for intervention. *Journal of Reproductive and Infant Psychology*, **6**, 23–39.

Nightingale, F. (1979). *Cassandra*. (Originally published in 1852). M. Stark, (Ed.), Old

Westbury, N.Y.: Feminist Press.

Nilsson, S., Mellbin, T., Hofvander, N., Sundelin, Y., Valentin and J., Nygren, K.G. (1986). Long term follow up study of children breastfed by mothers using oral contraceptives. *Contraception*, **34**, 443–57.

Nisbett, R.E. (1972). Hunger, obesity and the ventromedial hypothalamus. *Psychological Review*, **79**, 433–453.

Niven, C. (1985). How helpful is the presence of the husband at childbirth? *Journal of Reproductive and Infant Psychology*, **3**, 45–53.

Niven, C. (1986). Factors affecting labour pain. Unpublished doctoral thesis, University of Stirling.

Niven, C. (1988). Labour pain: Long term recall and consequences. *Journal of Reproductive and Infant Psychology*, **6**, 83–87.

Niven, C. (1992). *Psychological care for families: Before, during and after birth.* Oxford: Butterworth Heinemann.

Niven, C. (in press). Coping with labour pain: the midwives' role. In S. Robinson and A. Thomson (Eds.).

Niven, C. and Gijsbers, K. (1984). Obstetric and non–obstetric factors related to labour pain. *Journal of Reproductive and Infant Psychology*, **2**, 61–78.

Niven, C. (1986). Factors Affecting Labour Pain. Unpublished doctoral thesis. University of Stirling.

Niven, C. (1985). How helpful is the presence of the husband at childbirth? *Journal of Reproductive and Infant Psychology*, **3**, 45–53.

Niven, C. Coping with labour pain: the midwives' role. In: S. Robinson and A. Thomson (Eds.). *Midwives, Research and Childbirth. Volume 3.* London: Chapman and Hall. In press.

Nolen–Hoeksema, S. (1987). Sex differences in unipolar depression: evidence and theory. *Psychological Bulletin*, **101**, 259–282.

Norbeck, J. and Tilden, V. (1983). Life stress, social support and emotional disequilibrium in complications of pregnancy: A prospective, multivariate study. *Journal of Health and Social Behavior*, **24**, 30–46

Novello, A.C., Wise, P.H., Willoughby, A. and Pizzo, P.A. (1989). Final report of the United States Department of Health and Human Services Secretary's Work Group on pediatric human immunodeficiency virus infection and disease: Content and implications. *Pediatrics*, **84**, 547–555.

O'Hara, M.W., Neunaber, D.J. and Zekoski, E.M. (1984). Prospective study of postpartum depression: Prevalence, course, and predictive factors. *Journal of abnormal psychology*, **93**, 158–171.

Oakley, A. (1988). Is social support good for the health of mothers and babies? *Journal of Reproductive and Infant Psychology*, **6**, 3–21.

Oakley, A., Rajan, L. and Grant, A. (1990). *Social support and pregnancy of obstetricians and gynaecologists.* **97**, 155–62.

Office of Population Censuses and Surveys. (1989). *Mortality statistics, 1986,* London: HMSO.

Olasov, B. and Jackson, J. (1987). Effect of expectancies on women's report of moods during the menstrual cycle. Psychosomatic medicine, **49**, 65–78.

Orbach, S. (1985). Accepting the symptom: A feminist psychoanalytic treatment of anorexia nervosa. In D.M. Garner and P.E. Garfinkel (Eds.), *Handbook of psychotherapy for anorexia nervosa and bulimia.* London: Guilford Press.

Orbach, S. (1986). *Hunger strike.* London: Faber and Faber.

Organizational Psychology Research Report No. 1. University of Stockholm.

Orth-Gomer, K. and Unden, A.-L. (1990). Type A behavior, social support, and coronary risk: Interaction and significance for mortality in cardiac patients. *Psychosomatic medicine,* **52**, 59–72.

Orth-Gomer, K. and Johnson, J.V. (1987). Social network interaction and mortality: A six year follow-up of the Swedish population. *Journal of chronic disease,* **40**, 949–957.

Osborn, J.E. (1986). AIDS, social sciences and health education: A personal perspective. *Health education quarterly*, 13, 287–299.

Oxtoby, M.J. (1990). Perinatally acquired human immunodeficiency infection. *Pediatric Infectious Diseases Journal*, 9, 609–619.

Oxtoby, M.J. (1991). Perinatally acquired HIV infection. In P.A. Pizzo and C.M. Wilfert (Eds.), *Pediatric AIDS* (pp. 3–21). Baltimore, MD: Williams & Wilkins.

Padian, N.S., Shiboski, S.C. and Jewell, N.P. (1991). Female-to-male transmission of human immunodeficiency virus. *Journal of the American Medical Association*, 266, 1664–1667.

Papanicolaou, G.N. and Traut, H.F. (1943). Diagnosis of uterine and cervical cancer by the vaginal smear. London: Commonwealth Fund.

Papiernik, E., Bouyer, J. and Drefus, J. (1985). Risk factors for preterm births and results of a prevention policy. The Hagenau Perinatal Study 1971–1982. In R. W. Beard and F. Sharp (Eds.) *Preterm Labour and its consequences. Proceedings of the thirteenth study group of the Royal College of Obstetricians and Gynaecologists.* Manchester: Richard Bates.

Parlee, M.B. (1982). Changes in moods and activation levels during the menstrual cycle in experimentally naive subjects. *Psychology of Women Quarterly*, 72, 119–131.

Parry, B.L., Berga, S.L., Kripke, D.F., Klauber, M.R., Laughlin, G.A., Yen, S.C. and Gillin, J.C. (1990). Altered waveform of plasma nocturnal melatonin secretion in premenstrual depression. *Archives of General Psychiatry*, 47, 1139–1146.

Passannante, M.R. and Nathanson, C.A. (1985). Female labor force participation and female mortality in Wisconsin 1974–1978. *Social Science and Medicine*, 21, 655.Peterson, J.L. and Marin, G. (1988). Issues in the prevention of AIDS among Black and Hispanic men. American Psychologist, 43, 871–877.

Persky, V.W. Kempthorne-Rawson, J. and Shekelle, R.B. (1987). Personality and risk of cancer: 20-year follow-up of the Western Electric study. *Psychosomatic Medicine*. 49, 435–449.

Peterson, J.L. and Marin, G. (1988). Issues in the prevention of AIDS among Black and Hispanic men. *American Psychologist*, 43, 871–877.

Pettingale, K.W., Morris, T., Greer, S., and Haybittle, J.L. (1985). Mental attitudes to cancer: An additional prognostic factor. *Lancet*, i, 750.

Pettingale, K.W., Philalithisa, A., Tee, D.E.H. and Greer, S. (1981). The biological correlates of psychological responses to breast cancer. *Journal of Psychosomatic Research*, 25, 453–458.

Phoenix, A. (1989). Influences on previous contraceptive use/non-use in pregnant 16-19 year olds. *Journal of Reproductive and Infant Psychology*, 7, 211–225.

Phoenix, A., Woollett, A. and Lloyd, E. (1991). *Motherhood, meanings, practices and ideologies.* London: Sage.

Pike, M.C., Henderson, D.E. and Krailo, M.D. (1983). Breast cancer in young women and use of oral contraceptives, a possible modifying effect of formulation and age of use. *Lancet*, 2, 926–930.

Piot, P. and Laga, M. (1989). Genital ulcers, other sexually transmitted diseases, and the sexual transmission of HIV. *British Medical Journal*, 289, 623–624.

Pivnick, A., Jacobson, A., Eric, K., Mulvihill, M., Hsu, M.A. and Drucker, E. (1991). Reproductive decisions among HIV-infected, drug-using women: The importance of mother-child coresidence. *Medical Anthropology Quarterly*, 5, 153–169.

Polivy, J. and Herman, C.P. (1985). Dieting and bingeing. A causal analysis. *American Psychologist*, 40, 193–201.

Poma, P.A. (1987). Pregnancy in Hispanic women. *Journal of the National Medical Association*, 79, 929–935.

Population Reports (1988). Oral contraceptives, *Population Reports* Series A number 7.

Population Reports. (1990). Voluntary female sterilization. *Population Reports*, series C, number 10.

Porter, M. (1991). Contraceptive choices: an exploratory study of how they are made. *Journal of Reproductive and Infant Psychology*, 9, 227–235.

Reading, A.E. (1983). The influence of maternal anxiety on the course and outcome of pregnancy: a review. *Health Psychology*, 2, 187–202.

Reading, A.E. and Cox, D.N. (1985). Psychosocial predictors of labour pain. *Pain*, 22, 309–315.Reamy, K.J. and White, S.E. (1987). Sexuality in the puerperium: a review. *Archives of Sexual Behaviour*, 16, 165–186.

Refield, R.R. and Burke, D.S. (1988, October). HIV infection: The clinical picture. *Scientific American*, 90–98.Refield, R.R., Wright, D. and Tramont, E. (1986). The Walter Reed staging classification for HTLV-III/LAV infection. *New England Journal of Medicine*, 314, 131–132.

Registrar General Scotland (1990). Annual Report. London: HMSO.

Reid, J., Ewan, C. and Low, E. (1991). Pilgramage of pain: the illness experiences of women with repetition strain injury and the search for credibility. *Social Science and Medicine*, 32, 601–612.

Rimer, B.K. (1992). Understanding the acceptance of mammography. *Annals of Behavioral Medicine* (in press).

Roberts, M.M. (1989). Breast screening: time for a rethink? *British Medical Journal*, 229, 1153–1155.

Robinson, J.O., Hibbard, P.M. and Laurence, K.M. (1984). Anxiety during a crisis: emotional effects of screening for neural tube defects. *Journal of Psychosomatic Research*, 28, 163–169.

Rodin, J. and Ickovics, J.R. (1990). Women's health: Review and research agenda as we approach the 21st century. *American Psychologist*, 45, 1018–1034.

Rodin, J. (1981). Social and environmental determinants of eating behavior. In: L.A. Cioffi, W.P.T. James and T.B. Van Itallie (Eds.), *The body weight regulatory system: Normal and disturbed mechanisms*. New York: Raven Press.

Rodin, J. and Ickovics, J.R. (1990). Women's health: Review and research agenda as we approach the 21st century. *American Psychologist*, 43, 1018–1034.

Romans-Clarkson, S.E. and Gillett, W.R. (1987). Women who regret their sterilization: developmental considerations. *Journal of Psychosomatic Obstetrics and Gynaecology*, 7, 9–17.

Rosenberg, L. (1987). Case-control studies of risk factors for myocardial infarction among women. In E.D. Eaker, B. Packard, N.K. Wenger, T.B. Clarkson and H.A. Tyroler (Eds.), *Coronary heart disease in women*. New York: Haymarket Doyna.

Rosenberg, L., Kaufman, D.W., Helmrich, S.P., Miller, D.R., Stolley, P.D. and Shapiro, S. (1985). Myocardial infarction and cigarette smoking in women younger than 50 years of age. *Journal of the American Medical Association*, 253, 2965–2969.

Rosenman, R.H., Brand, R.J., Jenkins, C.D., Friedman, M., Straus, R. and Wurm, M. (1975). Coronary heart disease in the Western Collaborative Group Study: Final follow-up experience of 8 years. *Journal of the American Medical Association*, 22, 872–877.

Rosser, S.V. (1991). Perspectives: AIDS and women. *AIDS Education and Prevention*, 3, 230–240.

Roy-Byrne, P.P., Rubinow, D.R., Hoban, M.C., Grover, G.N. and Blank, D. (1987). TSH and prolactin responses to TRH in patients with premenstrual syndrome. *American Journal of Psychiatry*, 144, 480–484.

Royal College of Physicians of London (1991). Preventive medicine, a report of a working group. London: Royal College of Physicians.

Rubinow, D.R., Hoban, M.C., Grover, G.N., Galloway, D.S., Roy-Byrne, P., Andersen, R. and Merriam, G.R. (1988). Changes in plasma hormones across the menstrual cycle in patients with menstrually related mood disorder and in control subjects. *American Journal of Obstetrics and Gynecology*, 158, 5–11.

Ruble, D.N. (1977). Premenstrual symptoms: A reinterpretation. *Science*, 197, 291–292.

Ruderman, A.J. (1986). Dietary restraint: A theoretical and empirical review. *Psychological Bulletin*, 99, 247–262.

Ryder, R.W., Nsa, W., Hassig, S.E., Behets, F., Rayfield, M., Ekungola, B., et al. (1989). Perinatal transmission of the human immunodeficiency virus type 1 to infants of seropositive women in Zaire. *New England Journal of Medicine*, 320, 1637–1642.

Salmons, P.H., Lewis, V.J., Rogers, P., Gatherer, A.J.H. and Booth, D.A. (1988). Body shape dissatisfaction in schoolchildren. *British Journal of Psychiatry*, 153 (supp. 2), 88–92.

Sanders, D., Warner, P., Backstrom, T. and Bancroft, J. (1983). Mood, sexuality, hormones and the menstrual cycle. I. Changes in mood and physical state: Description of subjects and method. *Psychosomatic Medicine*, 45, 487–507.

Sarno, A.P., Miller, E.J. and Lundblad, E.G. (1987). Premenstrual syndrome: Beneficial effects of periodic, low-dose Danazol. *Obstetrics and Gynecology*, 70, 33–36.

Schachter, S. (1978). Pharmacological and psychological determinants of smoking. In R.E. Thornton (Ed.), *Smoking behavior: Physiological and psychological influences*. Edinburgh: Churchill Livingstone.

Schachter, S. (1971). Some extraordinary facts about obese humans and rats. *American Psychology*, 26, 129–144.

Schachter, S. and Rodin, J. (1974). *Obese humans and rats*. London: Wiley.

Scheeran, P., White, D. and Phillips, K. (1991). Premarital contraceptive use: a review of the psychological literature. *Journal of Reproductive and Infant Psychology*, 9, 253–269.

Scherg, H. and Biohmke, M. (1988). Association between selected life events and cancer. *Behavioral Medicine*, 14, 119–124.

Schmidt, P.J., Nieman, L.K., Grover, G.N., Muller, K.L., Merriam, G.R. and Rubinow, D.R. (1991). Lack of effect of induced menses on symptoms in women with premenstrual syndrome. *The New England Journal of Medicine*, 324, 1174–1179.

Schnall, P., Alderman, M.H. and Kern, R. (1984). An analysis of the HDFP trial. Evidence of adverse affects of antihypertensive therapy on white women with moderate and severe hypertension. *New York State Journal of Medicine*, 84, 299–301.

Schoenbach, V.J., Kaplan, B.H., Fredman, L. and Kleinbaum, D.G. (1986). Social ties and mortality in Evans County, Georgia. *American Journal of Epidemiology*, 123, 577–591.

Schonfield, J. (1972). Psychological factors related to delayed return to an earlier life-style in successfully treated cancer patients. *Journal of Psychosomatic Research*, 16, 41–46.

Schwyhart, W.R. and Kutner, S.J. (1973). A reanalysis of female reactions to contraceptive sterilization. *British Medical Journal*, 3, 220–222.

Scott, V. and Gijsbers, K. (1981). Pain perception in competitive swimmers. *British Medical Journal*, 283, 91–93.

Scott-Heyes, G. (1984). Childbearing as a mutual experience. Unpublished D.Phil thesis. New University of Ulster.

Scott-Palmer, J. and Skevington, S.M. (1981). Pain during childbirth and menstruation: a study of Locus of Control. *Journal of Psychosomatic Research*, 25, 151–155.

Search, G. (1988). *The Last Taboo: Sexual Abuse of Children*. Harmondsworth, Middlesex: Penguin.Sejwacz, D., Ajzen, I. and Fishbein, M. (1980). Predicting and understanding weight loss: Intentions, behaviors and outcomes. In I. Ajzen and M. Fishbein (Eds.), *Understanding Attitudes and Predicting Social Behavior*. New Jersey: Prentice-Hall.Shnall, P., Alderman, M.H. & Kern, R. (1984). An analysis of the HDFP trial. Evidence of adverse affects of antihypertensive therapy on white women with moderate and severe hypertension. *New York State Journal of Medicine*, 84, 299–301.

Schonfield, J. (1972). Psychological factors related to delayed return to an earlier life-style in successfully treated cancer patients. *Journal of Psychosomahil thesis*. New University of Ulster.

Schwyhart, W.R. and Kutner, S.J. (1973). A reanalysis of female reactions to contraceptive sterilization. *British Medical Journal*, 3, 220-222.

Scott, V. and Gijsbers, K. (1981). Pain perception in competitive swimmers. *British Medical Journal*, 283, 91-93.

Scott-Heyes, G. (1984). Childbearing as a mutual experience. Unpublished D.Phil thesis. New University of Ulster.

Scott-Palmer, J. and Skevington, S.M. (1981). Pain during childbirth and menstruation: a study of Locus of Control. *Journal of Psychosomatic Research*, 25, 151-155.

Search, G. (1988). *The last taboo: sexual abuse of children.* Harmondsworth, Middlesex: Penguin.

Sejwacz, D., Ajzen, I. and Fishbein, M. (1980). Predicting and understanding weight loss: Intentions, behaviors and outcomes. In I. Ajzen and M. Fishbein (Eds.), *Understanding attitudes and predicting social behavior.* New Jersey: Prentice-Hall.

Seligman, M.E.P. (1975). *Helplessness: On Depression, Development and Death.* San Francisco: Freeman.

Selwyn, P. (1991). Injection drug use, mortality, and the AIDS epidemic. *American Journal of Public Health*, 81, 1247-1249.

Shapiro, S., Venet, W., Strax, P., Venet, L. and Roeser, R. (1982). Ten to fourteen year effect of screening on breast cancer mortality. *Journal of the National Cancer Institute*, 69, 349-355.

Shekelle, R.B., Billings, J.H., Borhani, W.O., Gerace, T.A., Hulley, S.B., Jacobs, D.R., Lasser, N.L., Mittlemark, M.B., Weaton, J.D. and Stamter, J. (1985). The MRFIT behavior pattern study: II Type A behavior and incidence of coronary heart disease. *American Journal of Epidemiology*, 122, 559-570.

Shiloh, S. and Saxe, L. (1989). Perception of risk in genetic counselling. *Psychology and Health*, 3, 45-61.

Shumaker, S.A. and Hill, D.R. (1991). Gender differences in social support and physical health. *Health Psychology*, 10, 102-111.

Shuttle, P. and Redgrove, P. (1986). *The wise wound: The myths, realities and meanings of menstruation.* New York: Grove Press.

Skrabanek, P. (1989). Mass mammography: The time for reappraisal. *International Journal of Technology Assessment in Health Care*, 5, 423-430.

Slochower, J. and Kaplan, S.P. (1980). Anxiety, perceived control, and eating in obese and normal weight persons. *Appetite*, 1, 75-83.

Sloper, P., Knussen, C., Turner, S. and Cunningham, C. (1991). Factors related to stress and satisfaction with life in families of children with Down's Syndrome. *Journal of Child Psychology and Psychiatry*, 32, 655-675.

Social Trends (1986). London: HMSO.

Social Trends (1990). London: HMSO.

South, (1991, June/July). AIDS: The economic trauma. pp. 12-26.

Special Consulate to the Federal Minister for Community Services and Health on Women's Health (1988). *National policy on women's health: A framework for change.* Canberra: Australian Government Publishing Service.

Spiegel, D. and Bloom, J.R. (1983). Group therapy and hypnosis reduce metastatic breast carcinoma pain. *Psychosomatic Medicine*, 45, 333-339.

Spiegel, D., Bloom, J.R., Kraemer, H.C. and Gottheil, E. (1989). Effect of psychosocial treatment on survival of patients with metastatic breast cancer. *The Lancet*, October 14, 888-891.

Spiegel, D., Bloom, J.R. and Yalom, I. (1981). Group support for patients with metastatic cancer: A randomized outcome study. *Archives of General Psychiatry*, 38, 527-533.

Spitzer, S.B., Llabre, M.M., Ironson, G., Gellman, M.D. and Schneiderman, N. (1992). The influence of social situations on ambulatory blood pressure. *Psychosomatic Medicine*, 54, 79-86.

Stampfer, M.J. and Colditz, G.A. (1991). Estrogen replacement therapy and coronary heart disease: A quantitative assessment of the epidemiologic evidence. *Preventive Medicine*, 20, 47-63.

Stampfer, M.J., Colditz, G.A. and Willett, W.C. (1990). Menopause and heart disease: A review. *Annals of the New York Academy of Sciences*, 592, 193-203.

Stampfer, M.J., Willett, W.C., Colditz, G.A., Speizer, F.E. and Hennekens, C.H. (1990). Past use of oral contraceptives and cardiovascular disease: A meta-analysis in the context of the Nurses Health Study. *American Journal of Obstetrics and Gynecology*, 163, 285-291.

Starr, R.H., Dubrowitz, H. and Bush, B.A. (1990). The epidemiology of child maltreatment. In R.T. Ammerman and M. Hersen (Eds.), *Children at risk*, New York: Plenum.

Stein, Z.A. (1990). HIV prevention: The need for methods women can use. *American Journal of Public Health*, 80, 460–462.

Steinberg, M.D., Juliano, M.A. and Wise, L. (1985). Psychological outcome of lumpectomy versus mastectomy in the treatment of breast cancer. *American Journal of Psychiatry*, 142, 34–39.

Steptoe, A. (1984). Psychophysiological processes in disease. In A. Steptoe and A. Mathews (Eds.), *Health care and human behaviour*. Academic Press: London.

Stewart, B.E., Meyerowitz, B.E., Jackson, L.E., Yarkin, K.L. and Harvey, J.H. (1982, October). Psychological stress associated with outpatient oncology nursing. *Cancer Nursing*, 383–387.

Stoney, C.M., Davis, M.C. and Matthews, K.A. (1987). Sex differences in physiological responses to stress and coronary heart disease: A causal link? *Psychophysiology*, 24, 127–131.

Strickland, B.R. (1988). Sex related differences in health and illness. *Psychology of Women Quarterly*. 12, 381–399.

Sudlow, C. (1991). The contraceptive effect of breastfeeding. *The British Journal of Family Planning*, 17, 56–59.

Suls, J. and Fletcher, B. (1985). The relative efficacy of avoidant and nonavoidant coping strategies: a meta analysis. *Health Psychology*, 4, 249–288.

Tabar, L., Fagerberg, C.J.G., Gad, A., Baldetorp, L., Holmberg, L.H., Grontoft, O., Ljungquist, U., Lundstrom, B., Manson, T.C., Eklund, G., Day, N.E. and Petterson, F. (1985). Reduction in mortality from breast cancer after mass screening with mammography: Randomised trial from the breast cancer screening working group of the Swedish National Board of Health and Welfare, *Lancet*, i, 829–832.

Taylor, S. (1986). *Health psychology*. New York: Random House.

Telch, C.F. and Telch, M.J. (1986). Group coping skills instruction and supportive group therapy for cancer patients: A comparison of strategies. *Journal of Consulting and Clinical Psychology*, 54, 802–808.

Tennant, C., Bebbington, P. and Hurry, J. (1982) Female vulnerability to neuroses: the influence of social roles. *Australian and New Zealand Journal of Psychiatry*, 16, 135–140.

The Nation's Health. (1991, January). Novello cites research gap on women and AIDS. p. 4.

The Nation's Health. (1991, December). CDC announces expanded definition of AIDS. p. 4.

The Positive Woman. (1991, June/July). Recommendations for research on women and HIV infection. 5–8.

Thoits, P.A. (1986) Multiple identities: examining gender and marital status differences in distress. *American Sociological Review*, 51, 259–272.

Thomas, S.B. and Quinn, S.C. (1991). The Tuskegee Syphilis Study, 1932 to 1972: Implications for HIV education and AIDS risk education programs in the black community. *American Journal of Public Health*, 81, 1498–1504.

Thomas, H. (1985). The medical construction of the contraceptive career. In H. Homans (Ed.), *The sexual politics of reproduction*, Aldershot: Gower.

Thompson, L., Andersen, B.L. and De Petrillo, D. (1992). The psychological processes of recovery from gynecologic cancer. In M. Coppleson, P. Morrow and M. Tattersall (Eds.). *Gynecologic Oncology (2nd ed.)*. Edinburgh: Churchill Livingstone.

Turnbull, D. (1992) Psychosocial issues in implementing mammography screening in Australia. Unpublished PhD, University of Surrey.

Tymetra, T.J. (1990). Social and psychological repercussions of mass screening. In proceedings of the First World Congress "Safety in Medical Practice". Prevention and Compensation of Latrogenic Complications, Elisnore, Denmark, organised for ISPIC in collaboration with World Health Organisation Regional Office Europe, pp. 60–63.

U.S. News & World Report. (1991, December 16). Teenage sex, after Magic. pp. 90–93. World

Health. (1990, November–December). Paris declaration. 16–17.

Ussher, J. (1989). *The psychology of the female body*. London: Routledge.

Van den Akker, O. and Steptoe, A. (1985). The pattern and prevalence of symptoms during the menstrual cycle. *British Journal of Psychiatry*, 147, 164–169.

van Doornen, L.J.P. (1986). Sex differences in physiological reactions to real life stress and their relationship to psychological variables. *Psychophysiology*, 23, 657–662.

van Doornen, L.J.P. and van Blokland, R. (1987). Serum cholesterol: Sex specific psychological correlates during rest and stress. *Journal of Psychosomatic Research*, 31, 239–249.

Verbrugge, L.M. and Wingard, D.L. (1987). Sex differentials in health and mortality. *Women and Health*, 12, 103–145.

Vess, J.D., Moreland, J.R. and Schwebel, A.I. (1985). A followup study of role functioning and the psychosocial environment of families of cancer patients. *Journal of Psychosocial Oncology*, 3, 1–14.

Vessey, M. (1991). Breast cancer screening 1991: Evidence and experience since the Forrest Report. A Report of the Department of Health Advisory Committee. Trent Regional Health Authority: NHSBDP Publications.

Vessey, M.P., Lawless, M. and McPherson, K. (1983). Neoplasia of the cervix uteri: a possible adverse effect of the pill. *Lancet*, 2, 930–934.

Vinokur, A.D., Threatt, B.A., Caplan, R.D. and Zimmerman, B.L. (1989). Physical and psychosocial functioning and adjustment to breast cancer: Long-term follow-up of a screening population. Cancer, 63, 394–405.

Von Korff, M., Dworkin, S.F., Le Resche, L. and Kruger, A. (1988). An epidemiologic comparison of pain complaint. *Pain*, 32, 173–183.

Waldron, E. (1976). Why do women live longer than men? *Journal of Human Stress*, 2, 2–13.

Waldron, I. (in press). Gender and health related behavior. In D.S. Gochman (Ed.) *Health behavior: Emerging research perspectives*. New York: Plenum.

Waldron, I. and Lye, D. (1989). Employment, unemployment, occupation, and smoking. *American Journal of Preventive Medicine*, 5, 142–149.

Waldron, I. and Jacobs, J.A. (1989). Effects of multiple roles on women's health: Evidence from a national longitudinal study. *Women and Health*, 25, 3–19.

Walker, A. and Bancroft, J. (1990). Relationship between premenstrual symptoms and oral contraceptive use: a controlled study. *Psychomatic Medicine*, 52, 86–96.

Warner, P. and Bancroft, J. (1988). Mood, sexuality, oral contraceptives and the menstrual cycle. *Journal of Psychosomatic Research*, 32, 417–427.

Warr, P.B. and Parry, G. (1982). Paid employment and women's psychological well-being. *Psychological Bulletin*, 91, 498–516.

Warr, P. (1987). *Work, unemployment and mental health*.

Warr, P.B. and Parry, G. (1982). Paid employment and women's psychological well-being. *Psychological Bulletin*, 91, 498–516.

Warren, L.W. (1983). Male intolerance of depression: A review with implications for psychotherapy. *Clinical Psychology Review*, 3, 147–156.

Waters, W.E. (1970). Community studies of the prevalence of headaches. *Headache*, 9, 178–186.

Weidner, G., Sexton, G., McLellarn, R., Connor, S.L. and Matarazzo, J.D. (1987). The role of Type A behavior and hostility in an elevation of plasma lipids in adult women and men. *Psychosomatic Medicine*, 48, 136–145.

Weiner, H., Thaler, M., Reiser, M.F. and Mirsky, I.A. (1957). Etiology of duodenal ulcer: i. Relation of specific psychological characteristics to rate of gastric secretion (serum pepsinogen). *Psychosomatic Medicine*, 19, 1–10.

Weinstein, N. (1988). The Precaution Adoption Process. *Health Psychology*, 7, 355–386.

Weisman, A.D. and Worden, J.W. (1976–1977). The existential plight in cancer: Significance of the first 100 days. *International Journal of Psychiatry in Medicine*, 7, 1–15.

Weissman, M.M. and Klerman, G. (1977). Sex differences and the epidemiology of depression.

Archives of General Psychiatry, 34, 98–117.

Wellings, K. (1985). Help or hype: an analysis of media coverage of the 1983 'pill scare'. *The British Journal of Family Planning*, 11, 92–98.

Westoff, C.F., Bumpass, L., Ryder, N.B. (1976). Oral contraception, coital frequency and the time required to conceive, 16, 1–10.

Whitaker, A., Davies, M., Shaffer, D., Johnson, J., Abrams, S., Walsh, B.T. and Kalikow, K. (1989). The struggle to be thin: A survey of anorexic and bulimic symptoms in a non-referred adolescent population. *Psychological Medicine*, 19, 143–163.

Whitehead, M. (1988). *The health divide*. Harmondsworth: Penguin.

Whitely, B.E. and Schofield, J.W. (1986). A meta analysis of research on adolescent contraceptive use: Population and environment. *Behavioral and Social Issues*, 8, 173–203.

Wilkinson, R.G. (1990). Income distribution and mortality: A 'natural' experiment. *Sociology of Health and Illness*, 12, 391–412.

Wilkinson, R.G. (1992). Income distribution and life expectancy. *British Medical Journal*, 304, 165–168.

Willett, W.C., Stampfer, M.J., Bain, C., Lipnick, R., Speizer, F.E., Rosner, B., Cramer, D. and Hennekens, C.H. (1983). Cigarette smoking, relative weight and menopause. *American Journal of Epidemiology*, 117, 651–658.

Williams, S. (1992). Optimum forms of communication designed for women with abnormal cervical smears. Paper presented at Royal College of Nursing, Research Advisory Group annual meeting. Birmingham, UK.

Williams, R.B., Barefoot, J.C., Haney, T.L., Harrell, F.E., Blumenthal, J.E., Pryor, D.B. and Peterson, B. (1988). Type A behavior and angiographically documented coronary atherosclerosis in a sample of 2,289 patients. *Psychosomatic Medicine*, 50, 139–152.

Wilsnack, R.W., Wilsnack, S.C. and Klassen, A.D. (1984). Women's drinking and drinking problems: Patterns from a 1981 national survey. *American Journal of Public Health*. 74, 1231–1238.

Wilsnack, R.W. and Cheloha, R. (1987). Women's roles and problem drinking across the lifespan. *Society for the study of social problems*, 34, 231–248.

Wilson, J.M.G. and Junger, G. (1968). *Principals and practice of screening for disease*. Geneva: World Health Organisation.

Wingard, D.L., Suarez, L. and Barrett-Connor, E. (1983). The sex differential in mortality from all causes and ischemic heart disease. *American Journal of Epidemiology*, 117, 165–172.

Wolkind, S. and Zajicek, E. (1981). *Pregnancy: A psychological and social study*. London: Academic Press.

Woman Magazine. (1966). *The complete woman book of successful slimming*. London: Odhams Press.

Wooley, S.C. and Wooley, O.W. (1984). Should obesity be treated at all? *Association of Research into Nervous and Mental Disease*, 62, 185–192.

Woollett, A., Dosanjh-Matawala, N. and Hadlow, J. (1991). The attitudes to contraception of Asian women in East London. *The British Journal of Family Planning*, 17, 72–77.

World Health Organisation. (1985). *Women, health and development, a report by the Director General*. Geneva: World Health Organisation.

World Health Organization. (1990, October). AIDS and the status of women: Challenges and perspectives for the 1990s. *WHO Features*, No. 149, 1–3.

World Health Organization. (1991, November 11). World Health Organization says three-quarters of HIV infections transmitted heterosexually. *WHO Press*, Press Release WHO/54.

World Health Organization. (1991). Men and women sharing the challenge. *World AIDS Day Features*, No. 2, 1–4.

Worth, D. (1989). Sexual decision-making and AIDS: Why condom promotion among vulnerable women is likely to fail. *Studies in Family Planning*, 20, 297–307.

Worth, D. (1990). Women at high risk of HIV infection: Behavioral, prevention, and intervention aspects. In D.G. Ostrow (Ed.), *Behavioral Aspects of AIDS*, 101–119. New York: Plenum.

Wright, A.F. (1978). Surgical sterilisation in a New Town Practice. *Health Bulletin*, **36**, 229–234.

Wynn Parry, C.B. (1980). Pain in avulsion lesions of the brachial plexus. *Pain*, **9**, 41–53.

INDEX